A WARRIOR'S WAY

Insights for Cancer Patients,
Cancer Survivors and
Those Who Love Them

By John R. Cope
A Three-Time Breast Cancer Survivor

PREFACE

When you hear those three little words, "You have cancer," your life is forever changed. It may be better or worse, but it is never, ever the same. Cancer is affecting people's lives in almost an epidemic way. Yet the technological and medical breakthroughs for treatment are helping more patients to survive than ever imagined ten years ago. Today, recovery and survival are the expected outcomes if the cancer is detected at an early stage.

If more and more of us afflicted with cancer are surviving, what is the quality of our survival? Are we in denial, believing that cancer will never again touch our lives? Like some sort of mistake, something that we should never have been involved in? A quirk... a horrible accident?

Are we living in fear that the next ache or pain is a symptom of cancer's return? We do not talk about our fears. Instead we focus on other issues in our lives and bury fear deep within us. However, the fear never leaves us.

How do families, friends and co-workers cope with the situation? For some, there is no path to effectively dealing with cancer. Others find ways of coping successfully — of surviving — through strong family ties, through their religious beliefs or through their love and compassion.

Often people are at a loss to know what to say to a cancer patient. They want to offer compassion, but the right words and expressions of emotion are lost. Often, the reality of the cancer patient's condition reminds them of others they have known and perhaps lost. They find themselves avoiding any face-to-face sharing. That sharing is just too painful.

This book is about being a successful cancer survivor — in attitude, in action, in everyday behaviors. It's not a treatise on the "best" steps to take, because each of us must find our own "best" path. It is a composite of my three battles with cancer, and of surviving and learning and growing as a human being. I have also included insights and attitudes that other cancer patients and survivors have shared with me.

Cancer patients, survivors and the friends and family who offer love and support will find ideas, insights, behaviors and attitudes that can be adopted. I believe the reader will find a variety of useful support actions to take, to enrich the life of both the cancer patient or survivor and those who care. Each short chapter has a cancer survivor INSIGHT that reflects successful survival or support attitudes and actions each of us can take.

This book is not about the cancer treatments any of us should follow. It is not about religious precepts (there are virtually none included) nor is it about the correct behaviors to display when dealing with cancer. Most importantly, this book is not a "how-to" for being a cancer survivor, but more of the "WHY," that ever-important attitude of what it takes, at least from this author's experience, to be a successful cancer survivor.

As a three-time cancer survivor, I have more than sufficient experience to draw upon. In fact, it's far more experience than I wanted, but it's what I was given and as a result, I think I have something of value to say to others. I am a cancer survivor, thrice counted, and I am proud of being a warrior. This book is a part of creating something good from that experience.

Many people have expressed admiration for how I have been able to deal with cancer and carry on a professional life, and do so with good spirits and a positive attitude (at least most of the time). A big part of my successful survivor mentality are the attitudes I bring to the challenge. I am hoping that by sharing some of these ideas and convictions, it may help others to find their courage, their hope, and their personal path to being a successful survivor in a land where no one ever desires to journey. I have also included some humorous perspectives, because I believe a healthy sense of humor is essential to be a successful cancer survivor.

The reader will note that I never use the term "cancer victim." There is no place in this book, or in life, for being a victim. However, being a cancer patient includes the joys of chemotherapy, hormonal-therapy, radiation and other such self-induced poisonings to help eliminate the tumors that threaten our lives. I use the term "cancer survivor" frequently and liberally, because that's what I am and what cancer patients are becoming. We are all striving to survive the disease that threatens our existence.

But the real issue is, how do we survive cancer? Passively, like a victim in waiting? Or do we survive cancer by using the threat to help us listen to the voice inside, to live life to the fullest, to live and love as if our days are numbered, as if we had received a wake-up call?

I hope this book will be part of that wake-up call for those who need to listen to their inner voice, to decide to live their lives on purpose, because you still can. To not hear the wake-up call and continue to live life as it was before only denies the reality that your life has been changed, and you haven't been paying attention. This collection of affirmations, insights and attitudes is about making a choice to listen and to live on purpose.

I wrote this book for a number of reasons. Some of my motives were personal, shaped by my experiences in battling and beating cancer three times. I wanted to find a way to share my thinking and feelings — my survival mentality — with others, in the hope that it may inspire them and give them hope during their cancer treatment. During my own chemotherapy and radiation treatments, reading the stories of other survivors' courage, hope, and bravery in the face of overwhelming odds gave me the courage to be a warrior. It was what I needed to hear, to begin to think about my purpose for being on this earth. It was what I needed to read and hear to begin the journey of being a warrior, of being a successful and happy cancer survivor.

My journey is not over. The odds, according to my oncologist and the statistics from the American Cancer Society, are that I will battle cancer again. A fourth time seems unthinkable on an emotional level. It certainly is not something I want, but I must be prepared for the battle. It is a battle, not in a military sense, but in a focus of the physical, mental and emotional conviction to win. To lose is easy — just give up and let the cancer plant its victory flag. I refuse to give up and lose.

Through this book, I take one more step in planting my own flag as a warrior in the battle against cancer. This book is a statement of winning the battle and striving to achieve the highest quality of life I can. It's about living my life on purpose; of unconditional love, of appreciating the small things (and big things!) in life. It's about tasting the tears of joy and pain, of just being like other people, all the while knowing my cancer is only in remission and I must battle it again. I will battle it again, and I will succeed. That success is what this book is all about. That success is about life!

ACKNOWLEDGMENTS

Thanks to Betsy Collard, whose encouragement and support first cemented the idea of writing this book. She has been relentless in her encouragement and I thank her for that. To my lifelong friend, Larry Golda, who tried to teach me to write essays as my college instructor. His mentoring and encouragement through the years have motivated me to keep trying to learn to write those essays. To Annette Sabo, Kim McLaughlin and Myrna Daly, the illustrator, designer and editor who helped bring this book to fruition. Their work is also deeply appreciated.

Thanks to those who have been with me through my cancers and offered unconditional support, love, encouragement, and a good laugh or a kick in the pants when I needed it. They have helped me find ways to be a successful cancer survivor. My heartfelt thanks to Cam and Bill Braly, Rick Gilbert and Mary McGlynn, Steve and Chris Michaels and Larry and Edna Golda. To my son Jon, who never let me feel sorry for myself and is a hero to me in so many ways.

There are many, many others who should be thanked, but there is one person whose unconditional love, support, and more than anything else, her spirit, gave me the strength and courage to go on, when going on seemed impossible. My heartfelt thanks to my loving spouse, partner and number one champion, Kelly Jo Murphy. Without her, I would not be here today to write these words. We have many more Peter Rabbit adventures to begin...

TABLE OF CONTENTS

CHAPTER 1:
I DIDN'T KNOW
MEN COULD GET
BREAST CANCER

"Malignant neoplasm of the male left breast" was my clinical diagnosis, but for most men, it's an inverted nipple, sometimes with pain and sometimes without. Or it's a sore spot on the upper chest, as if you'd been poked with a sharp stick. Often the cancer goes undetected until the later stages, due to the masking of symptoms and lack of awareness of most men.

Typically, the discovery occurs during a routine examination or the concern is brought up as an afterthought, not the primary reason for the appointment. After all, men typically don't have mammograms or do self-examinations looking for bumps or tender spots. I have even heard some men say they "don't have breasts, they have chests." So much for the testosterone advantage!

Partly because male breast cancer is so rare, most men never have heard of it and, if they have, certainly don't discuss it. I personally had never heard of male breast cancer prior to my original diagnosis. After all, I was a guy, I was only 39 years old, an aging athlete, someone who took bumps and bruises in stride. The thought of having breast cancer was absurd. This lack of awareness means few men see a doctor before their breast cancer has advanced; consequently survival rate for men, according to the American Cancer Society, is much lower than for women.

Often a family history of female breast cancer will alert a male, but I was adopted and hence had no history to review. When I was first diagnosed (this was back in the dark ages, before the Internet and the World Wide Web) there was little information to be found about male breast cancer. The American Cancer Society, the hospital's library and other resources turned up very little, mostly just research documentation. Most of the cases were men in their seventies and eighties who had breast cancer along with other types of cancers.

I was the first male breast cancer patient my first oncologist, a physician who was nearing retirement, had ever treated. Since then, I have had three other primary oncologists, and one of the three had never treated a male breast cancer patient before.

According to the American Cancer Society, approximately one-half of one percent of all breast cancer diagnoses in the U.S. every year is of men — somewhere between 1,300 and 1,600 cases every year. Of that number, approximately 25 percent, or 400 men, will die. Males face a one in 800 chance of having breast cancer in their lifetimes. However, the disease will strike more than 175,000 women this year and kill about 25 percent or more than 43,000 women. Females face a one in eight chance of having breast cancer in their lifetimes. Male breast cancer is almost an anomaly.

The number of male breast cancer cases is on the rise, up from 800 cases annually a decade ago. There appears to be a high correlation between earlier detection and the rise in cases, but cancer researchers cannot confirm this. Historically, most male breast cancer diagnoses were in elderly men who had a number of other diseases and, consequently, the mortality rate was high. Today, with earlier detection and treatment, men's survival rate, like women's, is on the increase.

From a personal perspective, I recall two very different reactions from family, friends and colleagues. One, of course, was shock, concern, empathy and support. The other reaction, particularly from men, was something like… "Gee, I didn't think men got breast cancer, I thought that was just a female disease." The few cancer support groups that existed were exclusively female and not the most comfortable place for a male. I relied primarily on people close to me for my support group.

The good news is that treatment of male breast cancer is virtually no different than a woman would receive, where treatment processes are very well understood. Typically it begins with a biopsy to verify the tumor (or tumors) and the size, followed by surgery with a modified mastectomy (chest muscle removed in lieu of fatty breast tissue), removal of the cancerous lymph nodes, if any, and then on to the fun stuff of chemotherapy, radiation and recovery. Typically, no reconstructive breast surgery is required.

Much breast cancer, including men's, is spurred and fed by estrogen. Like women, whose tumors are "estrogen receptor positive," ongoing treatment for men, after chemotherapy or radiation, often consists of taking an estrogen "blocker" like tamoxifen or similar drugs. Unfortunately, there have been virtually no ongoing studies of their effects on men, due to the small number of male breast cancer patients. However, my oncologist assures me that males and females appear to react to the drugs in a similar fashion, including the side effects of weight gain and hot flashes.

I took tamoxifen for five years after my second round with cancer. The side effects I experienced were no different than women commonly report. Tamoxifen was discontinued (for obvious reasons — it failed to cause the desired effect of being an estrogen blocker) when I was diagnosed with my third cancer. However, I should say I believe it had a positive impact on my body's ability to "chemically block" itself from the estrogen positive receptors for five years.

Now, if you want an unusual combination in a man, mix equal amounts of kick-butt testosterone with an equal amount of sensitivity-type estrogen, throw in a little weight gain and those wonderful hot flashes and what do you get? A sensitive, macho kind of guy who is a little pudgy and has regular hot flashes! When I describe it that way, no wonder people think we're "special."

I don't often tell the world that I am a three-time breast cancer survivor. Who really cares? Besides, it only confuses people, who think, "Okay, you have two breasts but you've had breast cancer three times — what gives?"

For the record, my first breast cancer was in my left breast. The second breast cancer was two tumors, one in each lung. The third time, I had breast cancer tumors growing on my lymph nodes in my esophagus region. The ugly reality is that I fully expect to battle breast cancer again. The question is, where will it be next time? However, the good news is that breast cancer, in men or women, is well researched and understood. Improved methods and treatment approaches are used today, and the recovery rate continues to climb. In fact, many oncologists would say that breast cancer is the most predictable cancer to treat because it's so well understood and has been the focus of a great deal of research. Of course, the best news is that, if treated early enough, the recovery rate is very high.

INSIGHT: A WARRIOR'S WAY

Because the disease is so rare in men, most people are surprised to learn men can even get breast cancer. Many oncologists never treat a male breast cancer patient during their entire careers. Some men may feel embarrassed or awkward about having this predominantly female disease, but I assure you, this cancer will kill you just as it kills women. So, frankly, get over the embarrassment. Men can get breast cancer. Fight this disease, beat it, and survive! Count yourself as a member of a very small, elite group... because you are. You're "special."

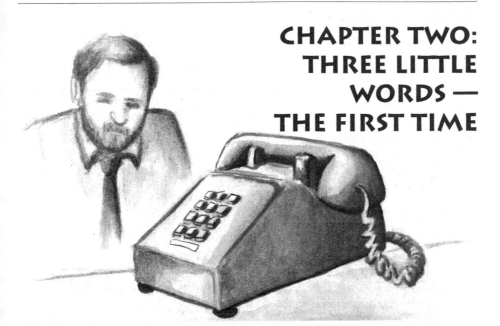

CHAPTER TWO: THREE LITTLE WORDS — THE FIRST TIME

There are moments in life that I will never, ever forget. Good or bad, the details remain rich in memory for a lifetime, always close to the surface: the day President John F. Kennedy died, when Martin Luther King was shot, and other events. Perhaps for other people, the birth of a child, losing a parent, getting married or even divorced are key memories.

These are milestones in our lives, benchmark points that we recall in minute detail: what we were wearing, the day or time, what the weather was like, who were we with and how we felt. These are common human experiences, usually triggered by some event that stimulates a flood of memories back to those moments. These shared experiences form a bond between people. All it takes sometimes is for someone to say, "Do you remember when you and I..." or "that crying sounds like our son when he was born..." or something similar. Bang! We're back in that moment as if it were yesterday.

For cancer survivors, the memory of hearing for the first time, "You have cancer," is never far from the surface. Cancer survivors can usually tell their stories in incredible detail — the moment or setting that changed their lives forever. I remember my first experience in hearing those three little words, "You have cancer" and in a level of detail that surprises me to this day.

In the summer of 1987, I was a training and development manager for a high-technology company in Silicon Valley. I was conducting sales training on weekends for telemarketers, and was dressed in a "casual Friday" style – knit shirt, jeans, tennis shoes, etc. During one Saturday session, I noticed that my left nipple area on my chest seemed to itch continuously, as if I had a mosquito bite.

At home, I removed my shirt and saw that my left nipple was inverted. I stood there, looking down at my chest: left side, nipple inverted; right side, nipple protruding; again... left side, right side, all the while wondering how this change had happened. I finally concluded that this was not normal, and since I didn't know what to make of it, I called my primary care physician first thing Monday morning.

I described the symptoms and, surprisingly, got an early appointment with no waiting. I thought at the time, "must be my lucky day." When I saw him, he examined me without saying much, other than he wanted to refer me to a surgeon for a biopsy to run tests. He assured me that it was probably nothing, but the tests from the biopsy could determine if it was something more serious than just an inverted nipple. I felt a sense of confusion more than anything else. If something was wrong, I thought, the area would be painful and this wasn't.

I was scheduled for the biopsy within a couple of days. When my wife Kelly and I met with the surgeon, he indicated that an inverted nipple was often associated with some diseases of a serious nature, including breast cancer. We discussed other ways I could have damaged the area — perhaps sports or car accident injuries. The biopsy was scheduled for the next day and the doctor would call me with the results a few days later.

I was planning to attend a special training program out of state the following week, so we agreed that he would call me there with the results. Kelly and I discussed the potential negative outcomes of the biopsy, but we were both optimistic that this little problem was nothing to worry about.

I was staying with close friends about a 40-minute drive from the training facility. I had planned to use the evenings to socialize and catch up on the events in our lives. I alerted them to the biopsy issue so they knew of the situation. Monday's events went smoothly and I anticipated that Tuesday would be the day of the telephone call from the surgeon.

The call came about 2:30 p.m., and I remember the doctor saying, "John, I have your biopsy report in my hand and I am sorry to tell you that you have cancer." He went on to say that he would like to do surgery as soon as possible, so the cancer wouldn't spread any further. He directed me to call his office when I returned from my trip and make the arrangements, and the sooner the better.

I vividly remember sitting by the phone after hanging up, feeling like I had just been run over by a freight train. I grew increasingly numb as my thoughts and feelings flooded through my brain. For the longest time I didn't move from my chair. My heart was beating as fast as I could ever remember and I realized I needed to leave the class and get into my car and go to my friends' house.

My first somewhat rational thoughts were hearing myself saying, "My God, I have cancer and I am going to die." The feeling overwhelmed me like nothing I had ever experienced. I felt helpless. I could not control the situation, and nothing would change the reality or reduce my pain. I must have said it more than twenty times, "I've got cancer." If I could think it and say it, perhaps I could deal with it.

I don't know how long I stayed in that office after I hung up the phone — 5, 10, 20, 30 minutes? I couldn't tell you to this day. When I decided to leave, I went back to the training room, gathered my things and whispered to the instructor that I had an emergency and had to leave immediately. I have no idea if anything I said was understandable.

I got in my car and drove to my friends' house. All the while, my head was racing with confusing thoughts, my emotions were spilling over, and all I could say out loud was, "My God, I have cancer, I have cancer, I HAVE CANCER!" The drive to their house was approximately 40 minutes and about 40 miles, mostly by freeway. Immediately after I arrived and to this day, I could not recall how I got there. I was in a sleep-like trance, a blackout of sorts, no short or long-term memory. It was as if I was desperately trying to get to a sanctuary to share my burden, to hear someone say, "You have cancer, but you'll be okay."

That was one of the strangest moments in my life: seemingly conducting business as normal (driving a car through traffic, on freeways, etc.) while I was having a complete implosion of feelings and thoughts that left me numb and yet hurting.

That evening, my dear friends provided me with love, hugs, laughs and compassion that allowed me to put this "cancer thing" into some kind of perspective, to begin to face the reality and to begin to think about the first steps to take.

The only thing worse that being told you have cancer is having to call long distance to your loved one with the awful news. No physical hugs, no arms and shoulders for crying. Such communication should only be done in person but this time it couldn't be avoided.

Kelly was on a plane to Oregon the next day, where we made up the time for hugs, and tears and shoulders to cry on. We were facing this together and we would beat this together.

The memory of being told I had cancer, in vivid detail and full color, is never far from the surface of my psyche. It never goes away.

INSIGHT: A WARRIOR'S WAY

Cancer survivors never forget hearing those three little words: the message and the associated emotions when they first learned of their cancer. It is a memory that can spring to life suddenly. Recognize this experience and its importance as a positive first step toward healing, recovery and surviving. Let yourself tell the story as often as needs to be told.

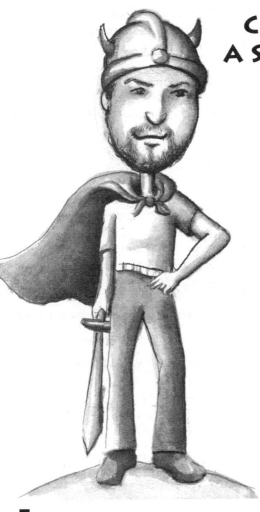

CHAPTER THREE: A SECOND BATTLE, AND I AM A SURVIVOR

In 1992, during my second bout with cancer, I knew it was going to be a very tough battle. In the first week, my hair began to fall out. The second week, my beard — my wonderful beard of twenty-plus years — came out by the handful... not a pretty sight. Soon I was totally bald, no eyelashes, eyebrows, leg hair, arm hair or chest hair. I looked like one of those Mexican hairless dogs — cute, but looking at me, you'd know there was something terribly wrong.

At work, I was gradually being excluded from meetings, and planning sessions for projects lasting more than a month were given to other people. I had all the "short-term" projects, meaning give John anything that we think he'll be around to finish. It was not an environment conducive to fighting cancer. People were more interested in bidding on my office with the window (to take it from me when I was too ill to work) than how I was doing. At times I felt invisible. Many people ignored me, avoided me and generally pretended I wasn't there. I became numb to their attitudes but, never, ever, to this day (obviously) have I forgotten how it felt.

After about three months of intense chemotherapy, I no longer had the energy to function in a full-time, demanding job. I was doing everything possible to continue working and making a contribution, but it was becoming more and more difficult. My professional self-confidence was eroding.

I knew I had stepped over the line into chemotherapy trauma one day when I left the office to drive home. I was tired, and as I tried to merge into the busy freeway traffic I realized my brain wasn't functioning fully and my normal quick reactions were slower. Trucks and cars seemed to zip by at warp speed as I tried to negotiate the short merge lane. I might as well have been driving a snowplow... I seemed to move at glacial speed while the traffic flow was almost impossible to deal with. I made it home safely, but I began to doubt my ability to function in this kind of multiple-task setting. I was beginning to lack the confidence to succeed.

As my chemotherapy progressed, I continued to lose more and more energy and consequently, my ability to think clearly. Even with a four-hour nap in the afternoon, I could not function at an acceptable level. It took more and more focus and energy to try to seem like a "normal" human being, let alone a cancer patient. I was beginning to question my ability to beat this cancer.

After all, I had a catheter sewn into my chest pumping chemotherapy directly into my primary blood-carrying veins, so it wouldn't cause permanent damage or leak outside the veins and vessels. Let's not forget the daily pills, and the weekly injections that would cause my hands to go numb and my veins to turn black like a heroin addict's.

So, what's the problem? Oh, that I was devoid of any hair, my skin color was like that sickly off-white computer printer paper and my clothes hung on me? Or that my thinking wasn't always clear or even intelligent? I had the physical and mental reflexes of someone who had mailed in their response and I could hardly prepare meals.

One day, about five months into a six-month chemotherapy regime, I woke up about five o'clock after a four-hour nap. Desiring to maintain my routine as much as possible, I went downstairs to begin dinner preparations. Our son was home from college so there would be three of us.

"Repeat after me, children, there are three of us for dinner with fours ears of fresh corn to divide among us. Okay, what's the correct number of ears of corn for each person?" I became confused and literally could not come to the correct amount. I struggled for the longest time until Kelly came home and helped me understand my confusion. Small wonder why I began to question my confidence to function anywhere near normal, whatever that was anymore. I tried to continue normal activities, but it was becoming impossible.

At this point, many people were encouraging me to put my faith in God ("He'll help you") or to "place your life in your doctor's hands, do whatever the doctors say," and one friend suggested a spiritualist, "to seek the faith... because at this point you have few options remaining." No wonder people were suggesting that I should put my fate into other hands. I was being poisoned to within an inch of my life, ON PURPOSE no less, my brain was groggy, my body was beaten up, I had become a sorry substitute for who I was... and yet, I still demanded to have a say in what happened to me.

Loss of self-confidence is inevitable when you look and feel like an old washrag. Throw in having the energy of a small towel and then imagine being snapped by the biggest bath towel imaginable every chemo or radiation day. Welcome to having the complete bath towel set, and you didn't even go shopping!

I began to focus on me — being healthy, beating cancer, fighting, winning, overcoming this horrible, suffocating disease that was killing me. I got angry, I had many private, out-loud discussions with myself about what was and was not going to happen to me. Damn it! I was going to win and beat this cancer — not my doctors, not God, not the chemotherapy, me!

Of course, I had no way of knowing what would happen to me. I knew from the doctor's diagnosis that I was at a crossroads of living and dying. Trying to think clearly when my brain was fuzzy from chemotherapy made everything confusing and anxious. I continued to believe, "I have to beat this, I refuse to let it take me. I have too much to live for and experience yet." Since I am not a religious individual, I saw no reason to take that path.

I don't have a label for the process or steps that occurred during the next few weeks of my chemotherapy. I know I focused internally on my desire and belief in my ability to beat cancer. I also know that a team of doctors guided my treatment using some of the most sophisticated chemicals and processes available. I even suppose a supreme power had a hand in the outcome. But ultimately, I believed that somehow, I was in control or at least doing my very best to try to be in control of my life.

Though I had come close to losing confidence in my ability to draw on my internal strengths, the same strengths that made me a unique individual, I still believed I played a key role in my survival. I still do today. I believe more than ever that I determined the outcome of my survival, not anything else. Survivors say, I beat cancer. Victims say, I didn't.

Be a survivor!

INSIGHT: A WARRIOR'S WAY

Surround yourself with positive forces — your family and friends, your faith, whatever positive forces you choose, and ask them to do whatever it takes to help you keep your self-confidence. Remember, it's you, not your doctors, not the medicine. Only you will BEAT CANCER! The help others provide is essential, but ultimately it comes down to your belief in yourself to be a successful survivor.

Enjoy the glow... and it's not from radiation or chemotherapy-induced sunburn trauma.

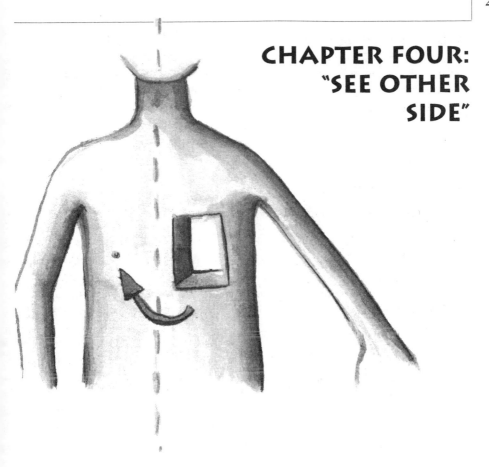

CHAPTER FOUR: "SEE OTHER SIDE"

Males with breast cancer are treated medically the same as women... almost. Biopsies, surgeries, mastectomies, chemotherapy, radiation... virtually everything is the same except, perhaps, for the issue of breast reconstruction surgery. This is where the two similarities end. Men simply do not have the societal, emotional, or physiological issues and needs with their "breasts" as women do. Yes, men have breasts, from a physical perspective, but losing one to a mastectomy has little emotional significance.

My first breast cancer resulted in a traditional mastectomy surgery, with a removal of the left nipple and related tissue, muscles, etc., leaving a clean but obvious scar from where my nipple was to my left armpit. Men often suffer from lack of muscle strength after surgeries like this, because most of the chest muscles are removed. Fortunately, I had a superb surgeon who carefully removed the tissue mass without removing unnecessary muscle.

My surgery was scheduled for an August morning, exactly one week before my 40th birthday. Talk about a birthday surprise! I was not to eat or drink after midnight the night before, as surgery was scheduled for early morning. Of course, I thought I would die of hunger when my surgery had a slight delay. Finally, after numerous complaints (actually, me whining), the attending medical staff gave me the pre-anesthesia about one in the afternoon. My spouse suspected the O.R. nurses got tired of my complaining and asking for scrambled eggs with bacon and toast every fifteen minutes.

My surgery was a simple one-day procedure with an overnight stay at the hospital. I had no complications and was able to return home the following day. Of course, my chest area was bandaged with enough gauze, tape and sterile covering to cover most of Nebraska. I had orders not to get the bandages wet for a few days, so showers or baths were out of the question. I would need to change the bandages frequently, however, during the first 48 hours at home. And I couldn't drive, since any stretching of either arm or torso rotation resulted in quick and lasting pain.

My dear friend Larry and his wife, Edna, were so concerned with my situation that they drove up to the San Francisco Bay Area to be with Kelly and me during this difficult time. On the day of my release from the hospital, Larry offered to take me home, which allowed Kelly some time to catch up on business requirements. On the way home Larry and I stopped for lunch as if nothing out of the ordinary had happened. "So, what's the lunch special today?" "Oh, by the way, how did that pesky surgery go?"

Sitting on my patio that afternoon, Larry and I, as longtime friends do, were joking and teasing about my surgery when it became time to change my bandage. This was my first opportunity to see where the surgery had taken place. I removed the bandage and even though I didn't expect to be surprised, I was! Looking down at my chest, besides the very obvious chest hair shaving marks, I was missing my left nipple. There was just a long, incision-like scar running from where my nipple used to be to my left armpit. The scar was barely visible, but I looked very, very, different. Good grief, I thought, I have a four-lane freeway heading across my chest and no rest area.

I'm not sure anybody gets accustomed to having body parts removed, and I was no exception. When I looked in the mirror, it was like I was seeing a set of eyes, with one eye closed and the other open, except it was my chest I was looking at. This has kind of a "pirate look," I thought, with a patch over one eye and the other eye open. I looked funny — off-balance and certainly different from before. I was not ashamed, but it upset the symmetry of my chest, so to speak.

I had no emotional issues about having my nipple cut off and the cancerous tissue removed. In fact, I was glad that the technology used by my surgeon could make such a difficult task appear so easy to do. My friend looked at me and made some jokes: "What's wrong with this picture?" and "Don't try this at home, kids," and we laughed and had a good time with my new physical appearance.

I looked down at my chest and decided I needed a little arrow saying "see other side" with the arrow pointing to my one remaining nipple. We began to laugh, and we each found comfort in joking about the situation. We were both glad it was just a little physical change in my appearance and not something fatal. This silly little observation got us started with a new set of creative ways to explain the obvious physical difference. Even to this day I still get a chuckle from friends. Of course, if you don't have a sense of humor and were offended by "see other side," well, I would rather be alive with a little geography change than not to be here. There's that attitude thing showing again...

I discovered early in my cancer survivor days that self-effacing humor, a tongue-in-cheek approach and a twisted wit and understatement made all the physical changes and challenges easier to take. As a male, losing a "breast" was not the path I would have chosen, but it is nowhere near as traumatic as a female faces. But finding ways to use humor to help yourself and those you love deal with the physical changes is just one of the keys to not being a victim, but a glorious survivor. If you don't believe me, see the other side of this chapter.

INSIGHT: A WARRIOR'S WAY

A sense of humor isn't mandatory for cancer survivors, but every single successful and happy survivor I have met has a sense of humor firmly in place. Laughter allows us to put things in perspective and ward off the ugly demons of this illness. Being a survivor with grace and dignity requires that we find humor in our physical changes. This is true for just plain getting old, as well.

CHAPTER FIVE: NOT A THIRD TIME

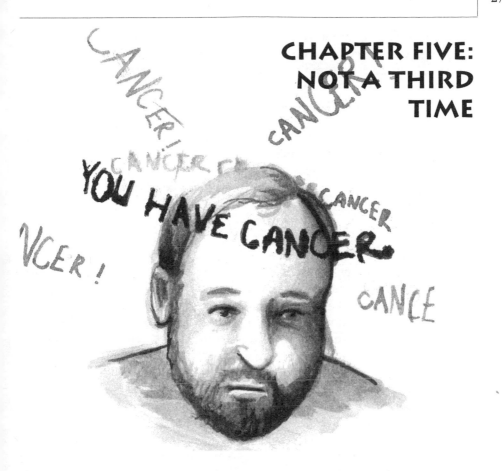

"**Y**ou have cancer." Those three words have changed the course of my life. Before, they were just words, but at the moment they mean everything. Nothing has prepared me for hearing them again, and there is nothing anyone can do or say to help me. I can't even help myself, but I know I must face the truth. I have to go it alone. Those three haunting words, YOU HAVE CANCER, scream at my very core. It can't be! It's not true! There must be some mistake! Why me? There are no answers. Only silence.

I am lying in a hospital bed, in the recovery area of the outpatient surgical wing, waiting and waiting with Kelly Jo. Dr. Asha, my pulmonologist, has just completed the initial surgical procedure, a radioscopy, essentially putting a fiber optic cable with a small optical lens up my nose and then down my throat.

The tension and anxiety are heavy. I try to joke to ease the tension in the room. "Hey Doc, check and see if I have any new email, while you're at it. Do

I get long distance phone service along with this wonderful adventure? Can I switch phone service providers and get frequent flyer miles?" She is mildly amused, jokes back and continues her procedure. I don't receive any email.

A radioscopy was selected as the best method to determine how big and where the tumor (or tumors) are in my air passageway. Rather than making an incision, it's a "non-invasive" method. A local anesthesia is used so I am as conscious and as alert as my brain allows me to be. Behind my facade of confidence in dealing with cancer lurks the "what if" question: Even though I try to think of something else, anything else, I keep asking myself, What if I have cancer again?

After the procedure, Dr. Asha comes into the room and asks how I'm doing and of course, as any good cancer survivor has learned to say, I reply, "I'm doing fine." In reality I am scared of the thoughts racing through my brain, let alone my heart. I don't even want to hear what she has to say. The look in her eyes says it all. She reaches out and grasps my left hand in hers. "Of course, we can't be sure until the pathology reports are completed after the biopsy surgery, but from what I saw, the tumors appear, well, they appear cancerous. I am so sorry it didn't turn out another way. I know you didn't want to hear me say that, but the tumors I saw..." She continues the detailed explanation, but I am still reacting to those three little words and I don't hear much else.

Tears form in my eyes as I close them tightly, as if to shut out the words. For a brief moment, I hear nothing; a huge emptiness surrounds me. I hear my own breathing and my pounding heartbeat. I begin to feel the warmth of my own tears as they run down my cheeks as the reality hits. I have cancer — AGAIN! Damn it, not again. My emotions bounce from anger to fear and back again.

Slowly, the fear subsides and I wipe away my tears. I have questions, but they can wait. I hug my wife and she hugs me back. For a moment, all is well. I feel safe, embraced in her love.

No one can prepare for this moment, for hearing those words a third time. But my entire life, and who I am, have prepared me to face this horrendous challenge once again, with all the courage I can muster.

My life is too full to have it threatened — again. Thoughts and feelings rush through me as I hear those words for the third time: You have cancer. Deal with it John, I decide. You don't have a choice.

INSIGHT: A WARRIOR'S WAY

You have choices in how you deal with cancer. You can feel sorry for yourself and become a victim, or you can take the survivor's path and face the reality: You have cancer. Nothing can ever prepare you for facing a diagnosis of cancer, but your life experience is your starting point. Surround yourself with people who love you — they will make everything so much easier. Ultimately, however, each of us faces cancer alone. You have choices to make.

CHAPTER SIX:
HURRY UP AND
WAIT

The ride home is full of questions and empty pauses. Sometimes the words don't come, and other times, I don't know what to say. At other moments I'm flooded with thoughts and feelings. My wife and I begin to ask the questions: Will I need radiation? Will it be chemotherapy again? How sick will I become? How soon will we begin? We talk of "we." We talk of "us." We don't use the words "you" or "I" by themselves, because now it's a "we" process. It's a battle Kelly and John will fight together. We share much, even the battle with the demons, but ultimately, each of us must face and fight cancer alone. Thank God she is there for me. It makes the alone part so much easier.

Biopsy surgery is scheduled for Monday, December 22nd. Dr. Asha's diagnosis was incomplete until a biopsy could be completed. Then I would know if it were a new cancer or, just as before, breast cancer. If it is a new kind of cancer, that could mean much trouble. If it's breast cancer once more, at least the treatment approaches are well known. I am secretly hoping it's breast cancer. I can handle that — it's the possibility of something new that scares me. I figure if I can beat this thing twice before, third time's a charm.

I am to be at the hospital early, around 8 a.m., with nothing to eat or drink for eight hours ahead of time. Of course there's a schedule change and my surgery is moved to later that afternoon. Oh great, by the time they get around to me later that afternoon, I could be dead of starvation... right in a hospital surgical department. Never mind cancer... how about feeding me while I wait, damn it! My pleas are ignored, and I get a sip of water every hour.

My wife and I talk, read magazines and phone our son. Other patients are coming and going in the area adjacent to me. Some sound okay and some sound like they are dying. God, I don't want to hear their moans. I have stopped asking when I'll get into surgery, because nobody can give me an answer. We watch TV and let the time pass as it will.

Our son is home, on the final day of his Christmas holiday with us. He's due to catch a flight out of Portland around 5:30 p.m., and a friend will take him to the airport. I feel bad that I didn't even get to hug him before he leaves. We talk, we say I love you to each other, but no father-son hug. In the back of my mind, a fear grows: What if you never return from surgery... and you didn't even get a chance to hug him again? It must be the lack of food that's toying with my mind.

I'm elated when the surgical nurses come for me around 5 p.m. "Finally, I'll get something to eat!" I hug my wife and she retreats to the hospital library to do more research on the kinds of cancers it could be. Meanwhile, the pre-operation anesthesia begins to take its toll. Slowly, I drift off into a near sleep.

Here's the part I can't understand: I'm lying there, drugged and sleepy, and the surgical team introduce themselves to me. I struggle to keep my eyes open as they say, "Mr. Cope, Hi, I'm Nurse Sally, I'll be assisting Dr. W tonight." Through my fog, it sounds more like, "Hi, I'm Sally, I'll be your waiter this evening. Tonight's special will be cancer identification, with just a small amount taken for biopsy purposes. We'll leave the rest inside of you. After the surgery, you'll be moved to a comfortable recovery room with absolutely no view. Of course, you'll still be hungry, but you won't really care. Eventually, after what seems like an eternity, the doctor will come by and ask you how you're doing." (First-time cancer patients, please note: if you say, "Not well," they'll keep you prisoner and feed you Jell-O or soup broth. If you say, "Hey! I'm doing great," they'll usually let you go home and eat real food.) After her introduction, I don't even get to order from the wine list before losing consciousness from the anesthesia.

Afterwards, as the anesthesia wears off, the pain begins to emerge. Good heavens, have they left an instrument in me? My chest and neck are very painful, so I ask for pain-killing drugs. Please note: doctors always seem to have "samples" to tide you over until you can get your prescription filled, so don't be shy about asking for some.

We are driving home again, my head is dizzy and I am hungry, although not as much as I was earlier in the day (strange how that works). I just want to eat a little something and go to bed. Being a surgical patient is hard enough, let alone dealing with cancer.

INSIGHT: A WARRIOR'S WAY

Fighting cancer is the hardest job you'll ever have. On top of the anxiety about the cancer, you'll face pain and discomfort, the side effects of treatment, and the "hurry up and wait" of appointments. During this difficult time, surround yourself with people who love you to help you through it. It also helps to develop your sense of humor, because you'll need it.

CHAPTER SEVEN:
TRUST YOUR
INSTINCTS

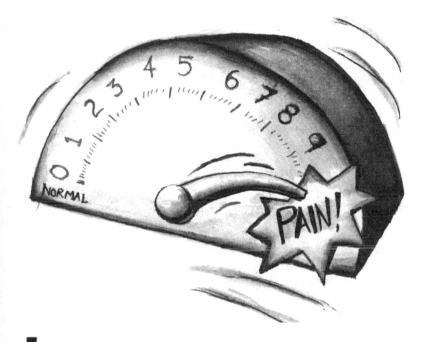

It's Christmas Day, and I wake up feeling like a big-rig truck ran over me in my sleep. I'm groggy, my head hurts, my throat screams at me, my temperature flips from hot to cold and back to hot again. Something's not right, but what could it be? After all, I just left the hospital less than three days ago.

I'm usually an avid breakfast eater, but today food sounds horrible. It's almost humorous, considering that I'd practically have killed for a hearty breakfast a couple of days ago, when my surgery was postponed for eight hours.

I get up, drink some juice and go right back to bed. Merry Christmas it isn't. I wake up a few hours later, drenched in sweat, the sheets soaked, my fever high, my heart pounding. My temperature is close to 103 degrees and I can't get cool.

Thirty minutes later, I'm freezing as my fever turns to chills. My temperature has dropped to 95 degrees. Can I put enough clothes on to stay warm? Do I have enough clothes to get warm? I'm somewhat delirious, or so I'm told later. Did you get the license number of that truck that just ran me over?

I'm confused, disoriented, my fever is doing back flips. I crawl back into bed. Kelly asks me, "How bad is the pain?" using the hospital's 1-10 scale for determining pain level. Despite having a high tolerance for pain, I let her know this is a 9 + in pain measure. This is the most pain I can ever recall — ever, ever, and ever!

Kelly calls the clinic and asks to speak with the on-call physician. Shortly, the doctor returns her call. She describes my symptoms, the sequence of events, how many days since my surgery, etc., and the doctor — I'll call him Dr. Penicillin — says emphatically, "Get him in to the emergency room here at the hospital immediately and if you can't, call an ambulance." Kelly keeps her composure and attempts to get me out of bed, dressed and into the car as quickly as she can.

Over-the-top pain does have a benefit: it blocks any rational thought and removes any memory records, so I am relying on what other people tell me about my condition. In a word, I am "out of it."

We arrive at the emergency room and a nurse at the reception desk greets us. I give him my name and he immediately escorts me to a small room to review my medical situation.

It must be my lucky day! Walk in, no waiting, go to the head of the line, and in fact, I was even escorted. Nothing worse than those pesky long lines in the emergency room on Christmas.

In the examination room the attending nurse collects data and takes my vital signs. The doctor arrives, asks a few questions and then wants to see the surgical wound beneath the bandage. He removes the bandage and says something to the effect of, "Well, it looks like we have a nasty old staph infection... probably got it during surgery last Monday. I think we can fix you up and get you on your way."

Excuse me, but how in the hell does a patient get a staph infection from a state-of-the-art, absolutely sanitary, cutting-edge hospital? It just seemed that a hospital should be the one place you wouldn't get a staph infection, but later others commented that a hospital is the only place they've heard of someone getting a staph infection.

The ER doctor gives me an injection to numb the pain and, tough guy that I am, I immediately pass out. Kelly leaves the small room and watches from the outside window. The doctor and nurse clean the wound and then decide that penicillin is needed, and a lot. Workers bring in a fifty-five gallon drum, or so it seems, and hook me up, via IV, to the largest penicillin container in the free world. Before they are through, they give me over 600 cc's of penicillin. When I emerge from my state of avoidance of pain, I have to pee so badly, I can hardly wait. Six hundred cc's of penicillin will do that to you.

The doctor gives Kelly a prescription for enough antibiotics to supply a small hospital and I am wheeled to the door. Once again, Kelly takes me home. Though the pain is significantly reduced, I still want to know the license number of the truck that hit me. Kelly and I talk in the car but I am groggy. We arrive home and all I want to do is sleep. Hope Christmas was good for you!

You can begin to see the pattern forming here; twice this week I have gone to the hospital, had some procedure done (and we're not even treating cancer yet!), leave the hospital with much more pain than I started with, return home where all I want to do is sleep.

INSIGHT: A WARRIOR'S WAY

When your body isn't acting like your body, something is wrong. Trust your instincts. Know how your body reacts to your treatment. You are the key to managing your care. See a doctor immediately if the symptoms are unexpected or seem to be getting worse. Don't wait until symptoms get so bad that you get to go to the front of the line at the emergency room. Trust me, it's not worth it.

CHAPTER EIGHT:
I'M A REALIST —
IT'S THE ONLY
WAY TO SURVIVE

One of the experiences cancer survivors know all too well is seeing the faces and bodies of others going through cancer treatment and wondering, do I look that bad?

In my second battle with breast cancer, I remember meeting a young man during my chemotherapy treatments. Mark was a computer technician on medical leave for an advanced case of leukemia. Married less than one year, he was optimistic that he would beat this horrible cancer in his body and go on to have a family. I remember thinking to myself, "This poor guy. Bald as an egg, skin the color of typing paper, and so thin that his bones stick out."

We'd converse about a variety of topics during our weekly "drip-trip" chemotherapy — just a pleasant conversation during an otherwise horrific time of self-induced poisoning. He seemed to need someone to talk to about the way the chemotherapy was ravaging his body. Since I looked and felt like hell, I was a logical role model for helping him through this difficult time. I enjoyed his company, but occasionally he wouldn't be there on Tuesdays. Knowing there are many reasons why a session would be moved or canceled, I didn't think much about it.

Occasionally I would miss a session because my white cell count was too low and would require a medication to artificially elevate my count to an acceptable level for chemotherapy. ("Let's see," my body is saying. "No thanks, I'm at the bottom of the roller coaster and I can't go to the top right now, so I'll just stay here. But with an injection of the white cell growth drug, within 24 hours I'll be ready for another full-scale invasion of chemotherapy so I can roar down the other side of the roller-coaster hill to a new bottom!" Usually, the bottom was lower than the time before, but believe it or not, somehow I got accustomed to it.

After Mark missed his treatment a few times I commented to the nurse that I hadn't seen Mark for a few weeks and wondered how he was doing. She looked at me with a sad expression.

"Oh, you obviously didn't know. Mark is no longer with us; he passed on last week." The shock of learning that someone I didn't know very well (but knew very well), who was in the same boat that I was in (weekly chemo injections), and who also had hopes and dreams, and didn't beat the cancer, hit me hard. I remember closing my eyes and thinking, I have to remain positive, I can't let this cancer beat me and I don't want Mark's fate to be mine.

The thoughts and fears of living daily and weekly while battling cancer make one a realist. I thought I was already a card-carrying realist, but I came to learn I was still a novice in that part of life. Mark's passing was a soft but important wake-up call. I was changing quickly from a novice into a full-fledged, hard-core, don't-sugar-coat-the-message, give-it-to-me-straight, realist!

I decided then and there, there is absolutely no substitute for accepting and dealing with reality. Each of us must do it, in our own way and style, but any-thing less than honestly accepting and facing one's own situation is giving up control of your life. I was choosing to retain control of my life's experience, regardless of how unpleasant it was at the time.

INSIGHT: A WARRIOR'S WAY

Cancer survivors have experienced the reality of battling for our lives. We have our feet on the ground, and we are painfully aware of how frag-ile this life is. Don't ask us to deny reality — it's what has made us strong. We cannot ever give up being in control of our life... it's the only one we have.

CHAPTER NINE: MOM WAS RIGHT ABOUT CHICKEN SOUP

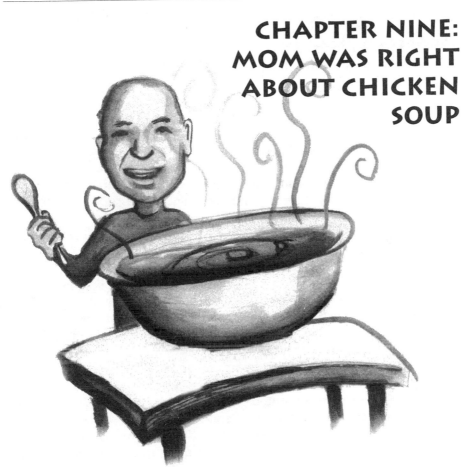

Most of us go through life eating and drinking anything we like. As we get older, we discover that spicy or "hot" foods often don't settle with us. The pharmaceutical industry has also discovered this, and is now selling us 50-year-olds all sorts of medications that will soothe the savage tummy or intestinal tract. We all carry antacids, "just in case." In fact, if you're a "baby boomer," you have already discovered that antacids have replaced breath mints as something we never leave home without. (If we'd known we were going to live this long, we'd have taken better care of our ourselves, right?)

Along comes cancer and KAPOWW! Food doesn't smell like it used to, doesn't taste like it used to and eating can be downright disgusting, if we can eat at all. Any cancer survivor can relate the experience of not being able to eat certain kinds of foods, or how some foods were okay during the first three months but intolerable after that.

My son used to say, during his formative and constantly eating years, "Food's food, let's eat." Oh, how I wished that were true. Prior to my first cancer, I could eat anything I wanted and never seemed to gain weight or have any discomfort. Food was something to be relished and enjoyed.

During my first battle with cancer, even six months of chemotherapy had only a slight effect on my appetite or ability to eat most foods. Especially spicy or rich foods might cause discomfort, but never for very long. I had no weight gain and after the treatment, foods returned to the taste of pleasure.

No weight gain was a surprise, since I had been taking large quantities of prednisone and would eat anything and everything in sight. Once I devoured an order of bread, butter and pasta at a restaurant and then proceeded to request a second serving. I have never done that before or since, but it shows the power of the little pills we take.

Since I'd had few problems during my first chemotherapy, I figured my second go-around of six months of chemotherapy would be a "cakewalk" (no pun intended). I couldn't have been more wrong. Whatever I thought I could eat, I couldn't. Does bland sound appetizing? Good, get used to it. Even water tastes different after awhile.

Suddenly everything I knew as okay foods were suspect. Everything gave me problems — too spicy, too hot, too rough, too _____ (fill in the blank) today. The next day, everything was different. My appetite was so picky and variable, I was suspected of being pregnant. Chinese pot stickers, for some strange reason, became a food staple for about a month. Then I couldn't stand the smell of them. Canned nuts were recommended for high protein, but soon I was gagging after a few of them. Soup was always good, but soup for every meal got a little old. Eventually even the thought of any kind of food made me queasy.

What happened? My oncologist had no definitive answer. Other cancer patients advised me to "get used to it — there's no good reason for it, it just happens." I began to truly listen to my body and discovered that one kind of food one week was wonderful but absolutely off the list the second week. No reason... it's just the way it was.

Over the course of my treatment, fewer and fewer foods sounded good. Between poor appetite and nausea, I lost close to 30 pounds. At about 150 pounds, my clothes hung on me like I was a super model, only I was not quite that skinny and I didn't walk funny and pout at the same time.

I made it through six months of extremely heavy chemotherapy, tolerated all the drugs and found ways to feed my scrawny body sufficiently to begin to return to a "normal" appetite. In fact, eating became an event and I enjoyed my regained ability to enjoy food without discomfort or nausea. However, I was on medication that had a minor side effect — weight gain. Not a lot of weight gain, just enough that dress slacks I had worn before chemotherapy wouldn't button less than six months later. My clothes went from "just hanging on me" to "sizes you once wore and can only dream about now."

I blamed the dry cleaners for shrinking my pants, especially in the waist, and then offering "tailoring" services. Oh, come on, I can see right through this ruse! Suddenly I was gaining not only weight but also inches. Soon my shirts, tee shirts, and even socks and handkerchiefs began to feel small. For an individual who never had to be concerned about gaining weight, suddenly having to watch "calories" was a strange experience.

About five months after my second chemotherapy I had a job interview in another city. I packed my suit — it had fit perfectly last time I wore it — and caught my flight. In my hotel room the next morning, as I was getting dressed for the interviews, panic struck. The jacket fit great, but I couldn't get the pants to button at the waist. It was like I was trying to put on a child's pair of pants. I must have tried that waist button forty times before facing the reality: I could not button my pants and breathe at the same time. Fortunately, my belt covered the gap and the zipper held. I interviewed all day, making frequent checks to be sure I wasn't coming undone. It was a tremendous relief to wrap up the interviews and change into another pair of pants, so I could breathe again. Oh, yes — I did get the job.

My third cancer, diagnosed in late 1997, was a tumor pushing against my throat and vocal cords. The carcinoma was located immediately behind my esophagus, or smack dab in the middle of my windpipe area, behind my breastbone. Receiving a radiation "nuke" every day for a couple of months seemed like an acceptable way to get this cancerous tumor obliterated. Compared to chemotherapy, radiation should have been much easier to tolerate. However, I was warned, it might cause "some small discomfort in eating or swallowing foods." Three days into the radiation treatment, I could hardly swallow water, let along food. By the fourth day I could barely swallow orange juice, leading me to conclude that I was in for one of the toughest times in my life. I believed the technical term is... screwed!

Each day, food became more and more difficult to swallow. Smaller bites seemed to work at first, but soon everything was painful. My esophagus seemed to be saying, "If you nuke me every day, I will refuse to allow even small particles of food to pass by without a swallowing reflex that will stop you in your tracks." Even with medication that numbed the esophagus, swallowing was so painful that all but a few foods were impossible. Even oral medications felt like I was trying to swallow golf balls.

Food temperature was also problematic. If the food was a little too hot or too cold, sorry Jack, you can't swallow. I tried to sneak ever-smaller bites through, but the esophagus guards on duty always caught me. God forbid I tried anything that hinted of spicy or acidic, like tomato soup. That was guaranteed to tie my entire body in knots. Not enough to just kill me, mind you, just enough to make me think I was on my way.

Then I discovered what mothers throughout the world have been saying for years. "Son, eat your chicken soup." Chicken soup was the only food my messed-up body would tolerate. In fact, it wasn't just any chicken soup, but specifically "Mrs. Grass's Chicken Noodle Soup," a dry soup mix with small noodles and just the right amount of chicken flavor. Though I had eaten it for years, I came to believe it was saving my life.

A good motto for eating chicken soup when you're not feeling well might be something like, "Chicken Soup: Cheer up! The chicken feels worse!" Of course, some days I felt more like the chicken.

My esophagus tolerated Mrs. Grass's Chicken Noodle Soup, and soon I was eating it all day long, in small amounts for breakfast, lunch, dinner and snacks. Though a one-food diet did get a little boring, I learned something that every cancer survivor needs to know: chicken soup is your friend.

INSIGHT: A WARRIOR'S WAY

Weight loss, weight gain, appetite swings, nausea...any or all can be part of cancer treatment. Expect it, and find whatever nourishment you can enjoy, or at least tolerate. Chicken soup, tacos, ice cream, or whatever else a cancer patient or survivor finds helpful, nourishing or at least non-painful will become a primary food staple. At times you can eat nothing without nausea or discomfort, so finding any food or drink that can be your friend is absolute goodness. As Mom used to say, chicken soup is your friend.

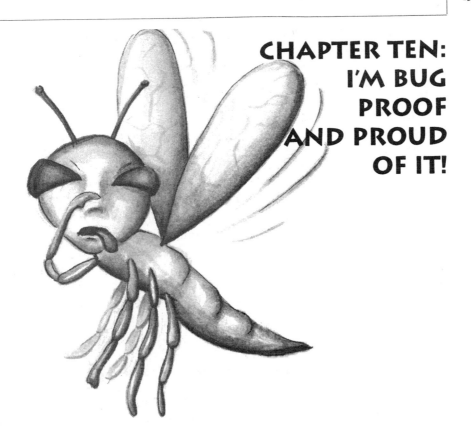

CHAPTER TEN: I'M BUG PROOF AND PROUD OF IT!

Ah, to enjoy a warm summer evening outdoors. Perfect, except for mosquitoes. My wife, Kelly, is "the" major mosquito attraction in the western United States. She's convinced that if there is just one mosquito within a hundred miles, it will detect her sweet smell and home in on her with a kamikaze death wish. She is almost guaranteed to get bitten, swollen and itchy.

Not me. A little-known benefit that most cancer survivors never share with "regular" people is that chemotherapy is the best bug repellent available. Think about it: if it makes your toenails ache when it's administered, leaves a metallic taste in your mouth like a chrome bumper, makes your hair fall out with just a smell, no wonder bugs think of you as the windshield of a '57 Buick Roadmaster.

Finally — a side effect of chemotherapy that's a perk. I can walk into the woods, hear that annoying little "bbbbbbbbbbbbbbbeeeeeeeeeeeeeeeeee" sound, feel them land and usually, but not every time, hear a little "P-yew" sound as they fly away. I'm bug proof and proud of it — a walking citronella candle, if you will.

Of course, the potential commercial value of this new bug repellent is probably low. Just imagine the field day marketers of a chemotherapy bug repellent would have. How about a new product called "Bite Me and Die," a truth in advertising approach to a chemo-based, citronella-flavored repellent? Or a spray version called "Bug-Off & Hair-Off Too!" The formula repels biting bugs and hair follicles as well — sort of a bald and bug-free look.

Of course, some of us have had the king of "bug killers." Having been shot with way too much radiation, I now glow in the dark, kind of like those backyard bug zappers. When the glow attracts the little biting critters, ZAP! POW! Once again, a little known side benefit of chemotherapy and radiation.

I know one thing for sure: Today I am cancer-free and proud of it. A lesser-known perk is that I am also bug-free. Eat your heart out, mosquitoes.

INSIGHT: A WARRIOR'S WAY

There are few "perks" to battling cancer, so if you've battled cancer and won, enjoy the sweet rewards of being a survivor, in whatever way those benefits come to you. Go ahead, take a walk in the woods. While the others are swatting away, you can enjoy the outdoors as a confident and bug-free cancer survivor.

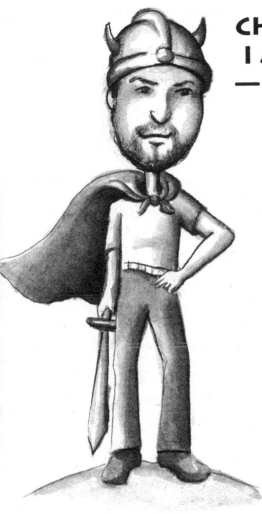

CHAPTER ELEVEN: I AM A WARRIOR — I AM A CANCER SURVIVOR

Battling cancer brings us in touch with our innermost thoughts and feelings. Sometimes it's overwhelming. There's a part of every cancer patient and survivor that would like to run and hide in a corner, covering our heads like a small child. We face the possibility of leaving our loved ones too soon, of giving up our careers prematurely and of not being able to fulfill our purpose for living.

For me, the term Warrior captures the essence of a healthy cancer survivor. Throughout history, "warrior" has been used to distinguish those who have battled their enemy and, through courage, strength and commitment of the heart, have prevailed. I invite you to join me in becoming a warrior in your own personal battle with cancer.

I AM A WARRIOR

I face the unthinkable and move forward...

I experience and embrace my feelings...

I awaken each day and determine to live my life with dignity...

I acknowledge my fear and uncertainty and choose to move forward...

I face my reality and accept the truth, but I continue to strive for victory...

I strive to be brave, even with tears clouding my eyes...

I face crises with honesty and resolve...

I believe in myself and my life's purpose...

I accept the unacceptable and move forward...

I AM A CANCER SURVIVOR

I face the diagnosis and make the best decisions I can...

I bravely accept the horrific daily medications and treatments, even when I want to stop...

I choose to receive the radiation treatments, even when one more seems like a hundred too many...

I acknowledge my fear and anxiety as I wait for the test results...

I help my loved ones accept and face the reality of battling cancer...

I see the future through our shared tears and never give up our vision...

I accept the unacceptable and strive to live...

I live life fully, with passion and appreciation...

I treasure each and every day of my life...

I face the battle by myself, but I know I am not alone...

I live my life on purpose, not knowing if there will be a next time...

I am given the gift of life, through the pain of cancer...

INSIGHT: A WARRIOR'S WAY

Cancer survivors — warriors — know that the next battle may come tomorrow or next year. We understand and accept the reality of fighting for our very lives. As warriors, we face the unthinkable and move forward with courage, whether we feel strong or fearful. All cancer survivors are warriors, and I am proud to be a warrior. Strive to be a warrior in your own way.

CHAPTER TWELVE:
THERE AREN'T VERY
MANY OF US
— THAT'S WHY WE'RE
SPECIAL

Each week the radio, TV and newspapers seem to have reports from the New England Journal of Medicine, the American Cancer Society or the "Anything and Everything Will Cause Cancer Clinic" with new data or research. I've become cynical as these new reports contradict last week's headline news. This week, pickles cause an increase in cancer and next week, fresh tomatoes will be linked with cancer cases. If I let my imagination roam, I'll soon conclude that EVERYBODY has or will get cancer.

From the American Cancer Society's 1999 statistics for breast cancer in the United States, as reported by the Associated Press, "Breast cancer was cited as the most common form of cancer in women, striking an estimated 182,000 U.S. women and 1,000 men each year. It is estimated that one of every eight women will develop the disease at some point. The disease kills about 46,000 women and 300 men a year."

Well, here's my attitude showing. This disease strikes one in eight women — one in eight. If women had a stronger political power base in this country, I'll bet we'd throw some serious resources at this problem.

How about men and breast cancer? Men are seldom mentioned as having the disease, but it's not just a female disease. One thousand men will get breast cancer this year in the U.S. and of that number, about three hundred men will die from it. That's a 30 percent mortality rate, a huge percentage.

If you research male breast cancer, as I have, you'll find studies from the American Medical Association and the American Cancer Society indicating that, of those one thousand men who are stricken with breast cancer, over 70 percent are over age 70 and have other significant medical problems. Of the approximate one-third that die each year, more than three out of four are over age 70.

I do not fit those statistics. I was diagnosed with intraductal carcinoma of the breast shortly before my 40th birthday in 1987, had breast cancer tumors in my lungs diagnosed on April Fool's Day, 1992, and in December 1997, was diagnosed with breast cancer tumors on lymph nodes in my upper respiratory tract. Many of my friends and work associates who have been diagnosed do not fit the statistical profile either. So, what are you to make of statistics?

No one is a "typical" statistic. If you get cancer — any gender, any age — all bets are off. You suddenly became a 100 percent statistic that you are a cancer patient. So, if you don't fit the statistical profile — and who does? — then develop the attitude that "I have cancer because I'm special ...just look at the odds." Why me? Who knows, and who isn't telling. You're the wrong gender, the wrong age, nobody in my family has had cancer, and so on. But now your only choice is to be determined and set your goal to be a cancer survivor. Show others that they're wrong, that you're going to survive and you're not finished living yet. You may have come up short on the "getting cancer" percentage, but you can become determined not to become one of those statistics. You are a warrior and a winner.

INSIGHT: A WARRIOR'S WAY

Attitude is everything. The more determined you are, the better. I absolutely, fundamentally believe that your attitude will contribute to your improving health and help your loved ones be better supporters and care providers. Your attitude will shape your response to the challenges you face as you move from "cancer patient" to "cancer survivor."

If you let statistical averages become your expectation, you'll become a statistic. Draw on your inner strength and develop the attitude that says, "It's not going to be me. I am the exception and not the rule. I'm special. Watch me survive and thrive."

CHAPTER THIRTEEN: THE DOG'S BEEN SLEEPING ON MY PILLOW AGAIN

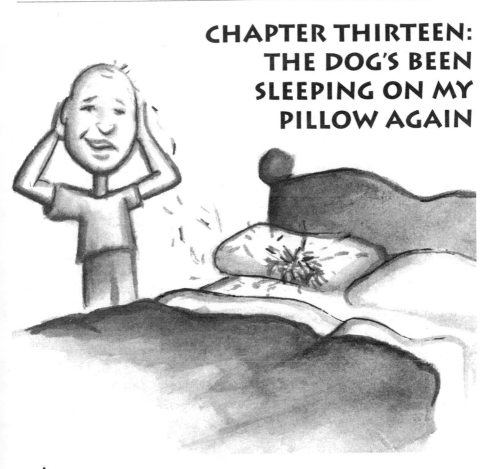

Ask any cancer survivor who has had chemotherapy or radiation about the experience of hair loss and be prepared to listen. Few events are as alarming or as terrifying as watching your own hair fall out, usually in great clumps or handfuls. It's a traumatic experience to reach out, grab some of your own hair and have it stay in your hand, leaving odd-shaped bald spots. It's bizarre, and it doesn't even hurt.

Admittedly, hair loss is a bigger issue for women than men. After all, it's fairly common to see men who are in their thirties, forties or fifties with that classic look known as male pattern baldness. One day during a boring staff meeting, I began to count the number of men in the room with a full head of hair. Among the staff of mostly men around the age of 50, there was only one of the twelve who had a full head of hair. The rest of us had only a historical resemblance to him. Seeing all that thinning hair, "U-rings" of hair and complete baldness, I suddenly realized I worked with a bunch of balding men. The few women on the staff had full heads of beautiful hair. (They could have shared some of that hair...) Few women go bald. Even grandma in her eighties, gray-haired and thinning perhaps, has a full head of hair. Grandpa's been bald for 40 years. But grandpa got there gradually, not over one weekend!

It's the sudden shock of having a normal-looking head of hair, along with eyebrows, eye lashes, arm hair, etc. one day, and the next, bang, you're going bald or have gone bald. It's very traumatic for anyone, but especially for women.

During my second chemotherapy, I was on a particularly heavy regimen of drugs noted for their ability to kill slow-growing cancer cells (and hair follicles too). Over one weekend, the hair loss got so bad I decided it was easier to just pull it out and shave my beard than to painfully watch it jump out of my body for a couple of weeks. We even videotaped me shaving my beard — my wonderful beard that I had worn proudly for most of my adult life. Needless to say, seeing myself with no beard for the first time in 25 years was a bit of a shock.

Next come the decisions: Should I wear a hat, should I not? How about a wig (especially appealing for women but not for a man... too many "rug jokes"). A scarf is nice this time of year (sure, August is perfect for those new summer colors). Perhaps nothing — just go out boldly and tell the world, "YES, I AM BALD AND BEAUTIFUL AND UNDERGOING TREATMENT FOR CANCER, GOT A PROBLEM WITH THAT?" Soon we calm down, become rational and figure out the best answers for ourselves.

But the body forgets that you're trying to poison it. Despite the daily chemical or nuclear assaults, it continues to attempt to grow hair. Nevertheless, the chemotherapy or radiation works its wonders and whatever body hair is produced gets promptly rejected. Over the course of a week or so, it is amazing how much hair you lose.

During my first chemotherapy, though I didn't lose my hair, it became very thin. One day I went to make the bed and there, on the bed, was a pile of little hairs — some short, some long, some straight, some curly, some dark, some lighter. Could this be from me? At that instant I decided to blame it on the dog. "Look at this, the damn dog's been sleeping in my bed again! What a mess! Where's the vacuum cleaner?"

And — we didn't even have a dog. So what! After the cancer treatment was over, I was prescribed a cancer preventive medication...with a side effect of "slight hair loss." Guess what? I still lose my hair, though at a much slower rate. Also, I still blame it on the dog, the same dog... which we still don't have.

INSIGHT: A WARRIOR'S WAY

Nothing — with the exception of being told you have cancer — is quite as traumatic as losing your hair. It happens quickly, it's not pretty and it's an affront to our self-image. Being bald — totally bald, including no eyebrows, eyelashes, etc. — tells the world, "look, here's a cancer patient." But remember, you're a cancer patient who is determined to be a cancer survivor. So face the world proudly, with or without a head covering. A sense of humor helps: When you see clumps of hair on your pillow, blame the dog... the invisible dog that's been sleeping on your bed again.

CHAPTER FOURTEEN:
WHAT DO YOU SAY
TO A CANCER
PATIENT?

"I have cancer" are the three scariest words anyone could think or say. What can your co-workers say or do to help you be strong? People who care about you are often fearful — your cancer, or any other life-threatening disease, reminds them of a family member, a friend, or stories they've heard. Some of the stories end positively... others don't.

What do I, as a cancer patient or survivor, need or want from my friends and colleagues? The answers are really very simple, but not so easy to do or to communicate.

During Breast Cancer Awareness week, I was asked to write a short article for a company newsletter about what cancer survivors or patients would like their friends and family to say or do. Here is what I wrote:

When you talk to me about my cancer...

I want you to let me know you care. Look me in the eye and say, "How are you feeling?" And wait for the answer. Let me tell you. I need that.

I want you to be strong and say, "I know you're going to beat this." Your strength stays with me.

Give me a hug of support, of caring. Hugs are good therapy for cancer patients.

I want you to laugh with me, because laughter makes the heart grow lighter. And share something funny or send me a funny get-well card. It really helps.

Keep me "in the loop" and informed of things that are happening. Tell me the latest gossip or news. I need something normal, because my life is not normal right now.

Don't say, "If there is anything I can do..." because it has no answer. Just be my friend and care, and be strong and laugh with me, and act normal... so I can feel normal, too.

INSIGHT: A WARRIOR'S WAY

Don't expect others to feel comfortable with your cancer. They are frightened, and they struggle with what to say. When your world is turned upside down, think upside down. Help others to feel comfortable, even when you aren't. It's one small step in regaining control of your life. Give others permission to ask you what you need.

CHAPTER FIFTEEN:
I LIVE MY LIFE ON
PURPOSE...
BECAUSE I CAN

I have chosen the words carefully: I choose to live my life on purpose. Here Is a simple explanation of the philosophy behind these words.

I live my life on purpose... today. I choose how I spend my energy and my time, my very precious time, because I know how fleeting it can be and I don't want to waste a single moment.

I choose what I do and what I stand for every day, because I can. I choose where I work, with whom I associate and the social events I attend. These are just a few of the simple decisions I make... because I can.

I have planned my hoped-for future to get more of what I want: my career goals, my financial security, my anticipated retirement and even where I live, because I want to achieve those goals on purpose... to maximize the experience of living today.

Twelve years ago, I received my first wake-up call. It came shortly before my 40th birthday — my first diagnosis of cancer. A harsh awakening for sure, but more of an inconvenience, a disruption and a nasty pothole on the road of life. In any given year, only one-half of one percent of all breast cancer diagnoses are of men. Get on with your life, I said, it was a mistake. It wasn't really a wake-up call, because I was choosing not to listen.

Four and a half years later, my cancer returned with a vengeance. I hit the wall again, a huge wall, and it gave me something back, a monstrous wake-up call. I was facing my mortality and I knew it. My immediate goal was to beat this cancer (again), but the prognosis was not favorable. I might not make it. Even my doctors were not optimistic. My mind retreated to some dark places attempting to imagine what I was facing. I wanted a future, but can I have one was the question before me.

Slowly, I began to appreciate the small things in life, everyday life, which now were so very precious, because I might not get the chance in the future. I wanted to live and I wanted to live on purpose — not by accident, but by being aware of my life, with every ounce of my being. I wanted to have the mundane days, the boring days, the over-stressed days, the too-much-time-in-traffic days, the lazy days, the rainy days and the days in paradise. I wanted to have more days, but I wanted to live them fulfilling my purpose in life.

Six months of chemotherapy, of carrying infusion pumps sewn into my body, of daily poisonings, of rushing to the emergency room, but I beat cancer, AGAIN! I was given the chance to choose to live my life on purpose, and it was time to start. Where I lived, what my lifestyle would be and how I spent my energy and time were all re-evaluated. I chose to make changes and I did... on purpose.

Cancer knows how to test one's purpose, determination and will to live like nothing else imaginable. I faced cancer a second time, and I was diagnosed with breast cancer a third time, ten years and a few months from the first diagnosis. Once the shock and horror wore off, I will never forget the feeling I had with the diagnosis... one of calm with little fear and only a few questions.

In light of my diagnosis, I asked myself if I was living on purpose. My answers gave me greater strength to battle this disruptive force in my life, once more. The answers showed me that today, my life is in greater alignment with my personal values, my beliefs and my purpose for existence than ever before.

My choices are purposeful. I am at peace with myself and my life because I am making the decisions... on purpose, because I still can. Twelve years after the first diagnosis, I have learned to live with cancer. Living on purpose prepares me to battle cancer yet again, because I know I will have to.

INSIGHT: A WARRIOR'S WAY

I live my life differently now. I feel its joy and beauty more intensely now. I appreciate each moment, because I live each day on purpose. Living life on purpose, by choice, enables us to control our destiny. Cancer survivors may not be able to control cancer, but they can choose how they will live their lives with cancer... and do so on purpose.

CHAPTER SIXTEEN: THE BEST DOCTOR ON EARTH

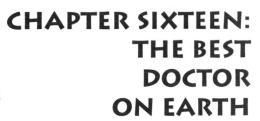

Cancer patients develop a close relationship with their oncologist(s) and the treatment support team. These dedicated professionals are committed to helping and supporting you during one of the most challenging periods in your life. What other situation has the following events: You get to watch someone poke needles into you, or fill your veins with poison or ask you to remain absolutely still while they go behind a lead wall and "nuke" you for what seems an eternity. Afterwards you're so appreciative of their work that you thank them sincerely for doing these things to you. It's a strange situation, for sure. Ask any cancer patient or cancer survivor about the meaning of trusting their oncologist.

I remember all of mine very well. My first oncologist, a distinguished-looking gentleman in his fifties, was associated with a number of research hospitals and had a gentle and reassuring manner about him that inspired immediate trust. He had that silver-haired look of experience and rock-steady emotions, never letting on what he was thinking or feeling. He simply conveyed a sense of control and authority. His staff worshiped him and other patients seemed to share my feelings of respect and trust.

My second oncologist was a foreign-born, U.S. trained and educated doctor who had the scientific competence of a research scientist, the knowledge of an experienced oncologist and the bedside manner of Attila the Hun. He wasn't mean, just matter-of-fact, always referring to the detailed clinical evaluation, rather than a more sensitive human approach. Though I respected his judgment and he certainly seemed up to date and extremely competent, I'll never forget our original conversation about my cancer (breast cancer tumors in my lungs). He looked directly at me and said, "Well, it doesn't look very promising. Either you'll be on your way to recovery in six months or you'll be dead." Okay, Doc, thanks for soft-pedaling it for me!

Toward the end of my six months of treatment, as I developed all sorts of complications my oncologist began to show a more sensitive side — or I began to see a very caring, human side behind the veneer of science. I suspect that doctors who are dealing daily with people who have cancer must develop thick skin to survive mentally and emotionally.

When my wife and I moved back to Oregon, I sought out an oncologist who came highly recommended and had a strong reputation in the community. I loved his bedside manner and his subtle but warm sense of humor. He was reassuring and comforting, traits I thought fit the field of oncology well. He treated me for almost five years during a remission between my second and third cancers. But when I needed to see him for my third cancer, I was told he was on a leave of absence and I would see a new doctor.

My current oncologist took over the practice, and I have found him to be extremely intelligent, personable, medically competent, practical in his communication and a genuinely nice person to be around. This has all the earmarks of his leaving the field of medicine, doesn't it?

During my third bout with cancer, my oncologist referred me for radiation in the hospital that his clinic is affiliated with. The hospital had a contractual arrangement with a medical group that specialized in radiation, pulmonary treatments, etc. It was convenient, as the radiation office was downstairs from my doctor's office. I was told that perhaps more than one radiation oncologist might treat me during the course of radiation, but I would have one primary and dedicated doctor.

I saw my original radiation oncologist just once before he transferred to another location. In his place, Dr. "C" would take over. So there I was, sitting in the examination room on the first day of radiation treatment, waiting to see my new doctor. The nurse left and I was passing time thumbing through magazines. After a slight knock the door opened and in walked my new radiation oncologist.

My immediate reaction — and this is strictly a guy thing — was, "Wow, what a babe! But where's my doctor?" She introduced herself as "Lori," the oncologist responsible for my treatment. My next reaction was, "Lady, do your parents know where you are? You're far too young to be a doctor — you're more like an attractive version of Doogie Howser (the TV show about a gifted young M.D. who was still in puberty)." My new oncologist had the looks and image of a TV soap opera doctor. You know the kind — very attractive, perfect smile, hair, dressed to the nines under her white lab coat... my goodness, I thought we were going to break for a word from our sponsors, soon.

When I recovered from the shock of having my doctor look younger than my own son, I found her to be a caring, smart and attentive physician. She knew what she didn't know and that's an important attribute when you're treating cancer. Since she was young in her career, her supervising doctor — the "senior actor" in this soap opera scene — was always nearby and coached her well.

Toward the end of my radiation treatment, she announced that she would be leaving the clinic to relocate to southern California with her husband. Her mentoring doctor took over my care and I never told her I would always think of her as the "soap opera babe doctor," not my radiation oncologist. I think it's best we keep this our little secret.

INSIGHT: A WARRIOR'S WAY

Oncologists come in all shapes, sizes, ages and colors — a truly diverse group. One thing that cancer survivors know, in their heart of hearts, is that their oncologist is the "best doctor on the face of the earth." This is the doctor who is trying to save my life!

It is critical that you have confidence in your oncologists and the team of professionals caring for you. If you don't have faith or trust in them, for whatever reason, and can't work out the differences, find a new doctor and team. You're worth it!

CHAPTER SEVENTEEN: ANOTHER MELTDOWN? GET OVER IT

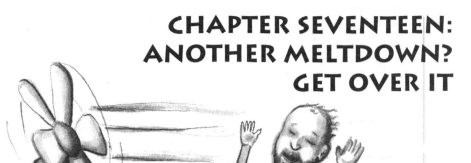

Modern cancer-fighting drugs save lives, reduce the chances of cancer recurring and, in general, contribute to an improved quality of life. As a cancer survivor, I have confidence that the medications I am taking are safe. But here I'm talking about side effects. Specifically, why do I have to experience these horrific, non-productive, sweaty, hot flashes on a daily basis?

Now, female readers will understand. I'm just sitting here, minding my own business, not running a marathon and suddenly the heat creep begins. On some days, they last less than 30 minutes and average about 125° Fahrenheit — just short of having your skin ooze off like in a class B horror film.

Other days, it's more like watching that same horror movie when the monster's face melts off... and I can't find a fan to cool down. My forehead sweats, always on the right side first, and then down to my lower face and over to the left side of my head. My body systems begin to scream, "MAYDAY, MAYDAY MELTDOWN, MELTDOWN, TAKE YOUR EMERGENCY POSITIONS" and the little fan in my hand is never quite enough.

Eventually I cool down, but my upper respiratory tract responds in a weird fashion, my sinuses think I'm having a major allergy attack, my eyes become fogged over and my hair looks like I just stepped out of the shower. My oncologist offers to prescribe a medication to minimize the symptoms, but that drug also has a side effect, causing a slowness of thinking. Thanks Doc, I'll pass. I think slowly enough already.

Believe me, guys, hot flashes are nothing to laugh at. Because I've been taking certain medications for years, I have learned to live with hot flashes, wipe my brow and get on with whatever I was doing. As a result, I have great empathy for women who experience them, but if I were to say something like, "Gee, I had another doozy of a hot flash this morning," people would look at me as if I had a third eye.

Cooling fans? I've tried them all. My loving spouse even bought me the little hand-held, battery-powered "cool fans," which help tremendously. I even have the large Mister Fan, which sprays water while fanning you. (You cool off, but look like you've been out in the rain. Not a good idea for the office. "John, thanks for the report, but why is the paper soggy?") I've tried them all — small portable fans, tabletop models, industrial strength floor stand fans with three-foot blades that you have to bring home in a pickup truck because they're so large. Sometimes even the huge ones with jet engine fan speeds don't help a single perspiration drop's worth!

When fans don't work, I go out to my vehicle and turn on the air conditioning full blast. Even better, I drive down the street with the windows rolled down, the air conditioning roaring and my head hanging out the window like an Alaskan sled dog in Florida. More than once I've had to change clothes because of meltdowns before going to work.

I've experimented with bandannas, gel-filled forehead coolers, chilled wash cloths, cool showers and a few other wacky approaches of mechanical ways to cool me down have been tried, usually with mixed results. What's next, moving to Alaska? The Arctic Circle? Everything's an option when I'm trying to avoid a public meltdown.

I have come to accept my condition, because I'd rather be here, enjoying life, than not to be here taking the medicine that causes hot flashes. And when I'm tempted to complain I remember what our friend Karen Wagner told me one evening over dinner: "Get over it, honey, and learn to accept those hot flashes — all of us women have."

The pearl of wisdom here is that every once in a while, even when I think I'm not feeling sorry for myself, I remember Karen's words: "Get over it, honey." It puts the challenges each of us face in perspective. I remind myself to drop the whining, complaining and self-pity. Warriors don't whine! For some people — and that includes all middle age women — hot flashes are just part of life. Things could be a lot worse. Ask any cancer patient or survivor!

INSIGHT: A WARRIOR'S WAY

Cancer teaches survivors many things, including empathy for others who experience difficult and perhaps life-threatening situations. Uncomfortable symptoms come with being a survivor. The real issue is about how open are we in accepting the personal responsibility of dealing with cancer. If each of us can accept what has happened, without blame or pity, then we can learn to be a warrior survivor. So get over it honey... and find ways to wear that sweat as a badge of courage.

HOT FLASH RELIEF

There is a naturopathic solution to hot flashes. Black Cohosh Root Powder (Cimicifuga racemosa), a dietary supplement, comes in a variety of pill forms and strengths. It is a root harvested in the Appalachian Mountains of Tennessee and sold through health food stores or the naturopathic section of pharmacies.

My oncologist recommended this solution, and I have found that, quite simply, it works! During the first two weeks of taking 200 mg pills, my hot flashes at first escalated in frequency and severity but then virtually stopped. I rarely have a meltdown — just an occasional sneaker hot flash to keep me humble, I suspect, but the intensity and duration are minimal.

CHAPTER EIGHTEEN: NOT ANOTHER BREAST CANCER BREAKTHROUGH REPORT!

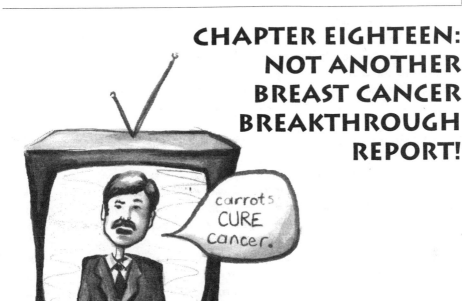

It must be television "sweeps month" or a radio ratings war, because I have heard more "breakthroughs in breast cancer research" announcements recently. Sometimes I want to just scream at all these stupid, childish teasers from the media under the guise of "keeping us informed."

Don't get me wrong. I am appreciative of legitimate reports on applied research efforts of intelligent and committed scientists and doctors, and I am hopeful their work will result in cures and preventive measures to control and eliminate cancers. However, I find little useful insight when a television news magazine story announces "steps each of us can take to prevent cancer" or the 6 o'clock news features "foods and vitamins that can help us prevent cancer," or the heart-wrenching story of "how a mother of two fights cancer and runs City Hall — story on our 6:30 news."

And there are the "teaser and filler" short stories that get squeezed into news programs, presumably gleaned from reputable sources. These have such headlines as "carrots can prevent cancer," or "drinking red wine can reduce the probability of cancer" or "eating red meat on Tuesdays, in even numbered months, if you're left handed and female, appears to cause an increase in cancer."

This kind of story, which always ends in a message of "hope and encouragement," is sensationalized, simplified, and ultimately, demeaning to cancer survivors. The approach is guaranteed to appeal to viewers, but real cancer battles and survivor stories aren't always so glamorous. Stories that end tragically are seldom reported, because they don't appeal to that sense of "hope" that media producers want.

When a famous television interviewer talked with a number of celebrities recently, I was shocked by the "spin" put on by the publicists. Here were actors, actresses, athletes, and other people in the public eye who had "battled" cancer. As each story unfolded, I was astounded by how each person had learned of their diagnosis, how they dealt with it ("bravely but didn't lose their hair"— as if they had a choice), and how much easier it was than they had anticipated. The "light chemotherapy" or "just a few radiation sessions did the trick" sort of explanation, "while continuing full time with their workload," sure didn't fit the reality of what fighting cancer is all about to most cancer survivors, including this three-time survivor. The glamorized stories, unfortunately, don't tell the real stories of men, women and children who have, perhaps, just a little more difficulty than "light chemotherapy."

There are notable exceptions. Scott Hamilton, the Olympic ice-skating champion and testicular cancer survivor, had a much different story. His story was about the pain, the agony and the physical and mental challenges he went through. He didn't pull any punches or give us the "sanitized" version. You knew he had gone through his own living hell and emerged, his will and desire pulling him along to recovery. His story was a real one, not packaged.

Hamilton also referenced his ongoing physical and mental challenges in being a successful survivor. He clearly demonstrated that the highs of returning to his calling (professional skating) are tempered by the reality of potentially facing cancer again. I salute him for his honesty and integrity and not succumbing to the temptation of the media's "make your cancer look like a challenge but not too difficult" way of thinking. And for goodness sakes, don't lose your hair!

The 1999 Tour de France winner, Lance Armstrong, became a media celebrity overnight with the story of his courageous battle with cancer. Like Hamilton, Armstrong's message was about the difficult challenges he faced and the personal commitment he made to be a survivor. His story was told with honesty and compassion in a no-nonsense manner.

This is not to imply that these celebrities didn't face real obstacles and tough times in fighting their cancer. I am sure they did. What I object to is the sanitizing of their experience in such a way that audiences begin to believe that cancer is no more difficult or life-threatening than the seasonal flu.

Every day, virtually everywhere, private and unknown individuals are conducting their own private battles with cancer. Some are succeeding and some are not. They are demonstrating courage, optimism and hope in their own battles against cancer. They don't need sugar-coated stories on television or the radio that trivialize their experience.

The truth is that many cancer survivors want to believe that cures and significant breakthroughs are just around the corner, because they need to have hope. I too want to believe that research breakthroughs are making a difference, but I have become jaded from the media's reporting every "study" as headline material. Even so, it hasn't stopped me from giving to the American Cancer Society on a regular basis.

Personally, I would like to see some balance and reality in what is reported, so people can be better informed. We cancer survivors would appreciate a lowering of the volume on the cancer breakthroughs.

INSIGHT: A WARRIOR'S WAY

Cancer survivors strive to be informed about their condition. However, we don't need more blaring television and radio announcements that only result in improving the media ratings and feeding the anxieties that may already exist about cancer. Scientific breakthroughs will come, but as a cancer survivor, I am living today, not in the future. I also change the channel regularly with my remote!

CHAPTER NINETEEN: THE OREGON DUCK FIGHT SONG BRINGS TEARS

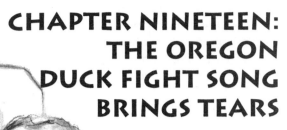

It was a clear, crisp day in September — perfect football weather. The sun was out but the feeling of fall was everywhere in Eugene, Oregon. We had come to my alma mater, the University of Oregon, to watch the "Fighting Ducks" battle the "Stanford Cardinal."

Crowds were filling the stands, the band members were tuning their instruments and the players were in the tunnel, waiting to be introduced. Everywhere one looked were the green and yellow colors of our beloved team. It reminded me of my graduate days at the U of O, sitting in the stands with my son, watching major college football action, usually in the rain, and enjoying the afternoon, regardless of whether we lost or won. It was the collection of the experiences, the emotion-filled afternoons, and all the colorful associations that brought back warm memories that afternoon.

The visiting Stanford Cardinals were introduced to the expected "boos," immediately followed by the introduction of the starting offense and defensive squads, welcomed by cheers and yells and whistles and of course, quacks from the plastic "quacker-maker" whistles. We were asked to stand and sing the National Anthem, which even on a bad day can make my emotions run high. This was a good day, and hearing the fans sing along with the National Anthem brought joy and a chill to my heart.

Then the Oregon Fighting Duck Band began playing the Oregon Fight Song as the players took the field. Somehow the music took me by surprise. I felt a lump in my throat and, slowly but surely, tears began to flow. As my heart raced, tears of joy flowed from this tough old warrior. It was great to be alive, it was wonderful to still be here and enjoy an afternoon of college football with my loving wife. It was great that I could still enjoy the smells, the sounds and the Oregon Fight Song... a song that invoked greater emotion than I had realized.

One is never quite ready for these unexpected and spontaneous bursts of joy and tears. It's an emotional rush that cancer survivors know well. I appreciate every day now, and never, ever, take it for granted. Little things like a familiar song or certain smells or feelings become the associated links to remembering how sick you were, and how sick and tired you were of being sick and tired.

Enjoy each day, for it brings wonderful new adventures, and who knows when those wonderful life memories will come flooding back, pulled out of your soul by a simple song. I think I want to come back for another game.

INSIGHT: A WARRIOR'S WAY

Allow your feelings to surface, and feel the feelings, no matter how difficult, because they are a part of who you are today. You are a survivor... rejoice in the fact you and I and thousands of other survivors are still here and living our lives. Football games may be won or lost, but successful survival is the ultimate victory.

CHAPTER TWENTY: YES, YOU COULD MOW MY LAWN...

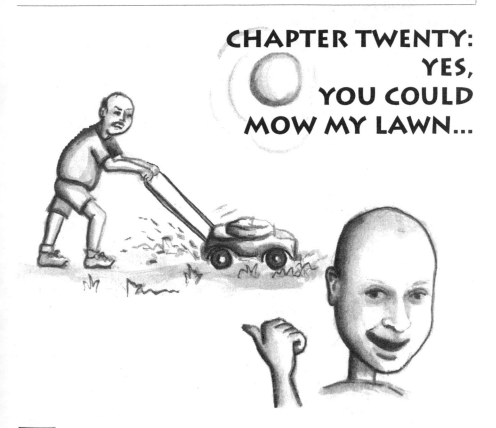

Through all three of my cancers, friends, family, co-workers, neighbors and others have responded with heartfelt concern and offers of help. These offers of "call me if I can do anything" or "if there is anything we can do, please don't hesitate to call" are expressions of concern by people who don't know quite how to express their true thoughts.

Cancer scares people, and the reality of someone they know being diagnosed with cancer only fuels whatever anxiety they already have. Yet, surveys consistently report that virtually every adult has come in contact with a family member, friend, or co-worker who has been diagnosed with cancer. This appears contradictory: on one hand, cancer is so prevalent that almost every adult knows somebody who has battled it. On the other hand, people don't believe (or don't want to believe) it can happen to them or someone close to them. When it does, reality becomes too close for comfort and they respond with vague offers that truly could not be acted upon.

I remember a time toward the end of my second cancer when my strength had been zapped, my brain didn't function clearly and fatigue was constant.

At the end of my seven-day chemotherapy cycle, my thinking would become crisper for a day or two before a new seven-day cycle began. This window of relief was all too brief before I repeated the chemotherapy cycle and became a slow-thinking bundle of duh! Again.

I was feeling particularly cynical, and probably a little sorry for myself during a conversation with someone I hadn't seen for awhile. We ended with an exchange of good wishes and then he said, "Now, let me know if there is anything I can do to help you during this awful time."

In my cynical way I responded, "Well, as a matter of fact, if you could mow my lawn, it would be much appreciated. It's very difficult for me to do that anymore." He looked at me as if I had asked him to be a bone marrow donor or join me in a bungee jump off a bridge. He was speechless for a moment, trying to determine if I was serious or just trying to be funny. He stumbled for a few seconds trying to find the right words, until I confessed, "I was just joking, I don't even have a lawn to mow. The homeowners' association takes care of what little lawn the complex has. I was just teasing..."

The look of relief on his face was worth a million bucks. On one hand, he was genuine in his concern and compassion for me and yet, he didn't really want to mow my lawn, even if I had one. I realize that my little teasing wasn't very nice but frankly, I was tired of what I perceived as hollow offers and empty words that would never be acted upon.

So, when someone asks "if there is anything I could do" I have a few other responses:

Yes, as a matter of fact, I could benefit from a complete blood transfusion, could you find time in your schedule?

Yes, as a matter of fact, my windows need cleaning and I can't do it, due to my weakened condition.

Yes, as a matter of fact, could you pay my monthly mortgage payment? It's so hard trying to work and do chemotherapy as well.

Yes, as a matter of fact, I do need an organ transplant... would next Friday work for you?

Yes, as a matter of fact, my gutters need cleaning and my house could use a coat of paint, thanks for offering.

Yes, as a matter of fact, could you go shopping for me and pick up some needed items, it's such an energy drain to fight traffic. I have a list prepared and thanks for offering.

Yes, as a matter of fact, I could use your help in moving this huge chair to the other side of the room, it's just that I don't have the strength I used to. Thanks for offering.

These last two are legitimate areas where many cancer survivors and patients could use help, especially during their treatment. These last two ideas and many other tasks require energy, focus, and stamina — something most cancer patients are lacking.

Most people don't expect to mow your lawn, yet they might offer if they knew it was a difficult task for you. If that's the case, go ahead and ask. Moving heavy furniture, even running some errands, are easy for people to do and would give them a great sense of helping and giving. Find some opportunities for those who truly wish to help you. You'll both be better for it.

Being the independent (read stubborn) sort, I didn't take advantage of all the help that was offered. In hindsight, the concerned and compassionate friends who offered to do something for me didn't experience the joy of giving of themselves. I also missed the opportunity to appreciate and thank them for their kindness. I will behave differently next time.

Besides, I am tired of mowing my own lawn...

INSIGHT: A WARRIOR'S WAY

People are anxious about cancer. They struggle to express their feelings about this disease, especially when talking to a survivor or a patient currently undergoing treatment. Often their words are sincere and well-intentioned but really can't be acted upon. Accept their good wishes — and offers, when you can — but don't be disappointed. Look for concrete ways they can fulfill their desire to help, and everybody will benefit from the love and caring.

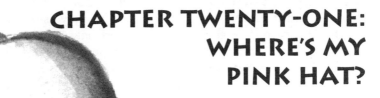

CHAPTER TWENTY-ONE:
WHERE'S MY
PINK HAT?

The Susan G. Komen Breast Cancer Foundation is a nationwide cancer fund-raising organization named for a courageous woman who fought and lost the battle with breast cancer. Each year, 98 local chapters from all over the United States stage fund-raising and awareness runs, walks, health fairs, marathons and whatever else the creative leadership can think of. Each year the Race for the Cure grows in participants and popularity.

Cancer survivors who participate in these run/walks get their own commemorative pink hat, signifying that the wearer is a breast cancer survivor. Family and friends who participate receive T-shirts with the name of the chapter and event date. Nothing is more inspiring than to watch a sea of pink hats moving down a city thoroughfare. In my community, the Race for the Cure is one of the largest organized running events of the year. A number of my female friends participate each year, sort of like a birthday of survival, and they always speak of the joy of the event.

A few years ago I decided that since I was a breast cancer survivor twice (this was before my third tangle with the stuff), I would contact the local chapter and ask about participating. You can imagine my astonishment when I was told that race participants are female and only females get the pink hats. "Well, what about men who are breast cancer survivors, don't we count for something?" I asked. She was at a loss for words but held her position that rules were rules and that was that. She did offer to allow me to participate in the event with other spouses, friends and family, but I declined.

The pink hat is symbolic of being a survivor, and I really wanted one, if for no other reason than to share the joy of being a survivor with so many others who had experienced a similar fate. I have counseled and provided help and support to numerous other breast cancer survivors (yes, they have all been women, but that is just a coincidence) and I thought the event would be inspiring. Watching the Race for the Cure on television is no substitute for the real thing. I had read accounts of a few men in other parts of the country who have participated in their local Race for the Cure and learned what it meant for them, personally, to be part of a sea of survivors, racing for the cure.

A few years later a woman wrote a letter to The (Portland) Oregonian questioning why men couldn't run in the 5K women's only Race for the Cure. Her close friend had just been diagnosed with breast cancer (for the third time) and she had seen men in the chemo rooms, and it didn't seem fair that they were prohibited from participating with other survivors in the main 5K race. Later I talked with the woman who wrote the original letter to the editor and that led to a local television station doing a spot on me and interviewing the race chair as well.

The race chair called me and offered to help me participate in the coed 1-mile walk. No, I answered, "I want to participate with other breast cancer survivors in the 5K, for the thrill and joy of the celebration of survival. I have no political agenda."

She agreed to let me participate in the 5K women's only race and personally helped me get registered. Later I received a phone call from one of the organizers of the Race for the Cure Survivor Luncheon, scheduled for the day before the race. The caller wanted to know if I would like to participate, with two other men, as a model in the fashion show. I agreed, and joined more than 800 people in a large downtown hotel for this beautiful, joyous event. Approximately 450 of the 800 attending were survivors. At the end, the house lights were dimmed and survivors stood and held lighted candles while the closing song was played. I don't think there was a dry eye in the place when the luncheon ended, including this old warrior's.

The next day, my wife and I drove downtown to participate with over 37,500 runners and walkers in the 5K Race for the Cure. The entry requirements have been changed from "women only" to "women only and all breast cancer survivors." The entire morning, before, during and after the race, other survivors wished me well. It was a thrill and a joy to participate and share in the celebration of being a cancer survivor with thousands of other survivors.

But what I am most proud of is, I finally have my own pink hat.

INSIGHT: A WARRIOR'S WAY

Cancer knows no gender boundaries, age boundaries, religious boundaries, sexual orientation boundaries, racial boundaries, or any other boundaries. When you have cancer, you join a special club, one you didn't ask to join, but which you cannot ever resign from. You're now part of a special family, called cancer survivors. Rejoice in that and wear any hat you choose.

CHAPTER TWENTY-TWO: MY SNEAKY LITTLE SECRET

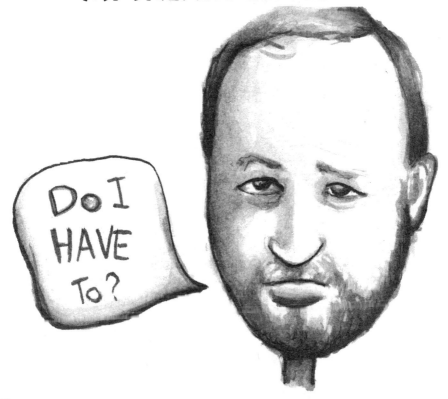

I'm going to share a little secret, one that sometimes works for me but lately seems to be less effective.

Let's face it, we cancer survivors sometimes get tired or lazy, or we simply don't feel like doing something. Maybe it's something as simple as taking out the trash or "while you're out, could you stop by and _____ " or any chore, big or small, that we simply don't feel like doing.

When you feel like that — a big lump on the couch — or you want to nap a little longer, or don't want to give up the TV remote, that's the time to pull out all the stops. Of course, you must appeal to someone's love, kindness, support, guilt or whatever emotion is at work in the situation, to pull off this escapade.

Simply follow this approach: Plant your tongue firmly in your cheek, create the saddest puppy dog eyes (the cocker spaniel look is the best) and the cutest look you can (guys, this may be a stretch) as you cock your head to one side. This is an important characteristic, so practice beforehand to get the full effect of sympathy (that's what we're going for here) as you say softly, "Do I have to??? Gosh, I have (or had) cancer..." letting your voice trail off in a "poor-little-me" fashion. Gazing to the floor with big, sad eyes earns extra points.

Had acting lessons? All the better. The important point is to use your situation, which is temporary, to get out of something you don't want to do.

I admit, I've had mixed results. At first my loving spouse, or others close to me, bought the act. "Oh, okay, you can sleep in a little longer, not do the shopping," or whatever chore or event I was dodging. Over time, their suspicions grew and now they're onto me, so choose your opportunities wisely.

However, every once in a while a new and unknowing individual would fall victim to my "Oh, I'd like to _____ but I have (or had) cancer." Once again my audience is falling over backwards in apology. This is not manipulation, but simply a golden opportunity to use your unfortunate situation to an advantage. Enjoy it while you can, because you're going to get well and won't be able to use this tactic forever.

Okay, now practice in front of a mirror by yourself, and the more syrupy your voice sounds, the better. Any questions? Good, go for it!

INSIGHT: A WARRIOR'S WAY

Hate chores? Use your secret weapon to full advantage. Play on the sympathies of loved ones and get them to prepare breakfast, run the errand or let you be lazy. You've earned it by having cancer. Enjoy this special status while you can, because soon you're going to be healthy and well and can't use this tactic anymore. Now it's your sneaky little secret as well, but I won't tell.

CHAPTER TWENTY-THREE: ANGELS ON EARTH

Oncologists and their staffs must be the equivalent of angels on earth. At times when I have felt so vulnerable, so in need of a kind word, a warm touch or a caring smile, an oncology staff member somehow seemed to know. In all my battles, I have never experienced a single staff member having had a bad day. Each employee always seemed to sense the mood and respond accordingly.

During my first cancer, I had chemotherapy sessions every Thursday afternoon after work (this schedule gave me three days to recover before returning to work). I remember the nurse who administered the chemotherapy. She was a kind and gentle person, explaining, almost in a tutorial manner, exactly how and why my fatigue would grow, why the veins in my hands were turning black, why the nausea was intermittent and what I should expect each week. Knowing what to expect always seemed to help.

Her manner was both a comfort and a source of strength to me. From her stories of other patients' battles I gained a great deal of insight into what motivated her to select this field of nursing, one that many would see as only about pain and suffering and death. She saw oncology nursing as helping people get well and resume their lives. She believed she had a greater impact on each patient's health than she would have in another role in another department.

During one of my chemotherapy sessions, a former patient poked her head into the chemo room to say hi, beaming with excitement. A follow-up exam had revealed that her cancer remained in remission, and she wanted to share the good news. The nurse was thrilled and later said to me, "That's why I do what I do and I want you to come back and visit me when you're well." I promised her I would, and I did.

During my second chemotherapy, visiting nurses came to my home to set up the catheter chemotherapy each week and to check on my overall condition. I was getting massive doses of chemotherapy, so they were careful to provide enough medical supplies — gauze, bandages, tape, iodine and the like. The hall closet looked like the supply depot for the local Red Cross. Each week it was a different nurse, yet each one shared the same positive qualities that made me feel good to be around them. They were always optimistic, always helpful and always genuine in their emotions. Their joy was in helping, in educating and probably most importantly, working with a cancer patient like me on a closer basis than they might otherwise have in a hospital setting. Bless them all!

The oncology nurses who administered chemotherapy in the clinic during my second cancer treatment were among the most courageous people I have encountered. Their workload seemed inordinately high, with many elderly patients who were not tolerating their chemotherapy well. Walking into the clinic, the smell of methotrexate, fluorouracil and cyclophosphamide seemed overwhelming and still affect me today when I am near any "chemo" room. Yet the oncology staff's helpfulness, their smiles, their spirit, always came through and you knew they were on a mission of compassion.

By the fourth month of my intravenous, catheter and oral chemotherapy, my skin was the color of typing paper, my eyes looked like I had been drinking alcohol all night and I didn't have one single hair on my entire body. I was losing weight, I had no strength and I hurt in parts of my body I never knew I had. Yet every week, the nurses would ask how I was doing, noting all the details in their notebooks and somehow, always made me feel a little more "normal" than when I walked in. They always genuinely cared and I'll never forget them for that.

During my third cancer, the daily radiation nurses and staff always went about the radiation procedures efficiently. It was a hospital setting, so one might expect a different kind of patient-staff interaction. The interaction was brief (you can only get "nuked" for a few minutes each day), but their attitudes and conversations were always pleasant and compassionate. Though the staff members changed roles frequently, every single one made the difficult radiation process much more tolerable. They all worked toward making the situation as normal as possible, in spite of how abnormal it was. I always thanked them each day for their help. Later I realized I was really thanking them for their commitment to helping.

During my first two chemotherapies, I received all my medications from the clinic and hospital pharmacies. In my third battle with cancer, the radiation was targeted at the tumors near my windpipe, hence the target zone was my upper-middle chest. Unfortunately, the radiation also "nuked" my esophagus. Within two weeks, I was experiencing so much pain that my liquid anesthesia medication wasn't adequate. My voyage into an ever-increasing depth of pain was just beginning.

I couldn't even sip water without a ten-minute acute pain reaction. As my doctors increased the dosage to combat this ever-increasing radiation burn on my esophagus, my local pharmacists were working to order, supply and dispense this critical medication. My biggest fear was that the pain would explode and I would run out of the medication or the pharmacy would be closed. On more than one occasion, I was in a state of panic, fearing that my medication wouldn't last until the pharmacy reopened.

These unsung heroes of the extended oncology team sometimes witnessed daily visits from me. I usually was in pain and probably not very nice to be around, yet they were always responsive, helpful and caring. I never expected to be recognized personally by any pharmacy staff, but day after day it was always, "Mr. Cope, how are you feeling today? Here's your medication..." I never could have made it through this critical phase in my treatment without their professionalism and help, and I just wanted to thank them one more time. Thanks!

INSIGHT: A WARRIOR'S WAY

Yes, they are all angels on earth, but ultimately, you are responsible for making sure you get the treatment you need. Be bold, be assertive, ask the questions and never take no for an answer. You deserve to have answers to your treatment questions. Possess the attitude that you are still in the driver's seat regarding your treatment, even if you feel awful. Remember, though, to always thank the angels on your team. They deserve it.

CHAPTER TWENTY-FOUR: "I CAN HEAR MY VOICE CRACK..."

My wife and I were having dinner one evening with a couple we met initially through business, but with whom we have much in common. "D" is also a cancer survivor and is currently facing another round of chemotherapy, less than two years after his first battle. As we were exchanging "chemo war stories" and sharing thoughts and concerns about living with cancer, the anxiety on his face was saying "Oh my God, here we go again..." Later that evening I was reflecting about another time Kelly and I had invited some friends over for dinner. When the subject turned to my three battles with cancer and the toll it takes, they were interested in what I was thinking and feeling during a particularly bad time in my second battle with breast cancer.

As I shared my thoughts and feelings, I probed a little deeper in my own mind and the emotions came flooding back. The fear of losing the battle, of dying, of not having the energy to take any more chemotherapy, even though I had to, were still very strong emotional issues for me. While not burying my emotions, I did keep these feelings buried a little deeper than I had realized.

As I told my story, my emotions erupted and I paused. "I can hear my voice crack," I said. I realized the pain and intense emotions associated with cancer survival can be brought back in an instant. A certain smell, a particular taste in the mouth, a person's voice or name, or even music or events can yank us back through time to those days when we had surgery, or were undergoing radiation or chemotherapy, or both. Regardless of how many years have passed, my experiences have not diminished in intensity; they are always there, always just an emotional flip of the switch away from surfacing. Experiencing these intense emotions from our battles with cancer can be healthy. We can never escape our experiences, but we can enhance the quality of the choices in our lives by remembering what we have been through. This context gives us the opportunity to enjoy going forward in a way only cancer survivors can know. "Hearing our voices crack" can be a healthy way to stay in touch with our emotional past.

INSIGHT: A WARRIOR'S WAY

Cancer survivors can never really bury (nor should they, I believe) the emotional experiences of battling cancer. While we don't dwell on those memories, they can surface in an instant. And you know what? It's okay that we remember. It can make us choose, on purpose, how we elect to live our lives today. We shouldn't bury those emotions and memories. "Hearing our voices crack" can be a vivid way of living every day on purpose. Can you hear your voice crack?

IN MEMORIAM

The "D" in this chapter was our friend, David Evans, who lost his battle with cancer in Portland, Oregon, December, 1999. David possessed a wicked sense of humor, a compassionate heart and is missed by his family and friends. David will always be remembered as a warrior for the courage, love and optimism of his spirit.

CHAPTER TWENTY-FIVE:
KEEP THOSE CARDS
AND LETTERS
COMING

love ya!

hello!

I miss you.

People struggle with what to say to a cancer patient, especially as the treatment continues and there is no "good news" to report. Often when the news is first announced, or if there is a surgery, people with good intentions will flock to the stationery stores to find a card with just the right message. During all three of my cancers, one of the major healing and motivating events was receiving cards, letters, poems, and sometimes handwritten, heartfelt messages from friends, family and other cancer survivors. All were important, and they all made a connection with me to aid in my healing.

During my first cancer in 1987, I was working for a major high-technology company in Silicon Valley. Since my cancer surgery was just days before my 40th birthday, it combined not one but two events: Happy "black-balloon 40th" and all the good-natured teasing that comes with it AND the "get-well, recover-soon-from-your-surgery" kinds of cards that people love to send to patients coming out of the hospital.

One of the cards began with "THIS PARTICULAR CARD, IN AND OF ITSELF, REALLY DOESN'T DO MUCH MORE THAN SAY HELLO." Inside was a drawing of a little dog with the caption, "BUT WITH A PAIR OF SCISSORS AND SOME TAPE, IT MAKES A NICE HAT FOR THE DOG." It was just the kind of card to cheer me up and bring a smile to my face. More important was that my friend took time to write a personal note, covering every square inch with her thoughts. Her words had a profound effect on me, and I believe the reader would also appreciate her message.

"Poor John, that was my second thought, my first was 'Oh no!' Why you, why me, why anyone? I just heard about you on Monday and still haven't totally absorbed the news yet. As you probably haven't either. I did beautifully the first few months — probably because I felt so awful the realities didn't penetrate. Or possibly, I was going through some form of denial. We all know people who have cancer, but it's never us! Finally, after 1 1/4 years, I can look at myself with a bit of objectivity and say —'Well, lady — you had cancer, you had it removed, you made it through that first critical year and if you make it to two years you've a 90% chance of getting home free.'

"Your emotions will do some crazy things to you now, John. But don't deny the legitimacy of those feelings — as crazy as they may sound. No one can understand them unless he's walked in your shoes. Mine ran the gamut from euphoria to deepest depression and despair. I've some books I want to recommend to you about getting well again, but please remember — if you throw them across the room sometimes in frustration and anger, you won't be the first one — I've done it and nearly broken a window. It's not easy to feel joy and hope and take control of your life when nausea shakes your body, you hurt, can't breathe and mostly feel very alone and scared. Somehow, in some way, at some times, they all have helped.

"If you feel like affiliating with a cancer support group, great! I didn't have the energy to drive to the hospital for the meetings — and part of me was frightened to be in a group of various stages of cancer — remission, recovery or terminal. I think the latter reason was the strongest. But it would have been an enormous comfort to talk to someone who knew what I felt. If you need me, I'm here — please don't ever hesitate to call if you'd like. Perhaps that's the one gift outside of prayers and thoughts that we 'c' people can give each other."

She included her phone number, adding that she would be away for a two-week vacation in the Caribbean "— a fantasy I never thought I'd do." And she recommended books that had helped her through her own ordeal.

"Oh my gosh — now I've used up all this space — A messy card but so filled with good thoughts and HOPE for you!"

I wrote back: Thanks for taking the time and energy and spirit to write your message. It made a difference in my life.

INSIGHT: A WARRIOR'S WAY

Making an honest and sincere connection with the cancer patient is the most therapeutic event that can happen. Sometimes the message is for ourselves and sometimes it's for the cancer patient or survivor. Sometimes it's for all of us. Humor is the path to healing so keep the "sad cards with flowery writing" to a minimum. Select something funny, or adapt what you purchased for the individual in a humorous way.

So keep those cards and letters coming, family and friends. The point is connecting from the heart, bringing a smile and letting the patient or survivor know you really care. It's all about healing.

CHAPTER TWENTY-SIX: THINK YOU'RE HAVING A TOUGH DAY? TRY THIS!

The wind is blowing in from the ocean, the sky is clear and sunny and there is enough of a "chill in the wind" that my loving spouse and I are settled cozily inside our motor home in the town of Ucluelet, on Vancouver Island, British Columbia. We're warm and comfy as the 5 o'clock news comes on the TV. After the local news items, the coverage switches to national and international news, including this story: "At the South Pole today, a physician, the only physician in the research facility, has found a lump in her breast and incredible efforts are underway to allow her to be own physician and patient."

My first reaction was, My God, not only is she dealing with the uncertainty of possibly facing cancer, but also she has to put on her professional hat (and clinical hat), and order the required equipment and supplies to be air-dropped onto the South Pole. Shipping, airlifting or evacuating from the South Pole in July were not options because it's too cold for equipment to operate out in the open. Landing aircraft was not possible either. An airdrop of equipment was the only option available.

Through the magic of technology, she could send her electronic images to a satellite to be downloaded to a university hospital for evaluation, but she couldn't be airlifted to the hospital due to Mother Nature's seasonal cycles. So, what's a doctor to do?

This woman was the only doctor in this underground settlement, measuring roughly the size of a football field. No one can leave the research facility for several months, due to weather conditions. She is not only the physician but the patient as well and she believes she has breast cancer. She intends to perform a biopsy by inserting a long needle into one of her breasts to get the tissue sample. Having had a similar procedure, which was one of the more painful experiences I can recall, I can't even imagine doing it on oneself. This procedure sounds like pulling your own wisdom tooth, but doing it slowly.

Suddenly, I am drawn to the big picture perspective... So, John, you think you had it tough? Imagine this woman — "pioneer" would be an understatement — who has discovered a lump in her breast. The good news is that she is a physician, the bad news is that she's the only physician for thousands of miles and due to the severity of the weather at the South Pole, no one can get in or out for at least three months.

Aside from the logistics of airdropping equipment or the technical aspects of beaming satellite images digitally back to a research facility in the U.S., imagine being a physician who is also the patient and facing cancer for the first time. Who helps you through this? Who can offer encouragement and guidance? Who provides the emotional support, the 'big shoulder to cry on' for the only doctor in the South Pole facility? Does the doctor give up her emotional needs in order to be seen by the community as a leader, not someone who needs support, care, compassion and big shoulders to be hugged into and to cry on? Where does her humanness come in?

I think of these things and imagine such a strong woman, a woman who is intelligent and brave and, probably, scared to death from what she is facing, to say nothing of what her family is going through, so far away. Imagine that phone call or whatever form of communication was used. Imagine the difficulty of words, of emotions, of not being able to connect, face to face, during such a difficult time.

At times like this, life issues come into perspective for me, for accepting and understanding and making things okay in my cancer-riddled world. I think of how I have accepted and dealt with the injustice of what has happened to me, and then I think of this physician/scientist/human being and what she is going through. It never ceases to make me humble.

It puts what I have experienced into a big, old, comfy chair and says to me, "You know, your situation was a tough battle, actually the pits, and you survived it. Now imagine what this person is going through." It is with this kind of personal perspective that I stand back and admire a tough survivor. Would I do what she is doing? Would I make the same kind of informed decisions and analytical requests? Would I hold myself together emotionally to cope with this entire situation? I hope so.

I rejoice to hear the follow-up news, that Dr. Jerri Nielsen, of Youngstown, Ohio, was evacuated safely from the South Pole on October 14, 1999, as temperatures plunged to nearly 70 below zero. Her original diagnosis was confirmed and she is expected to have a full recovery from the breast cancer and chemotherapy.

This is a survivor I would like to meet and talk with. I would like to hear her tell her story. This is a survivor I would like to understand what and how her thinking guided her through this tough situation. No "training or simulation" prior to the South Pole expedition could have prepared her for this. I would love to find one, just one, simple survival key to strengthen my own attitude about dealing with cancer.

When I pause to reflect, I come to the realization that her actions are the one simple thing to learn from. She has given me one more sign to learn from. It's all about hope and courage and moving forward when it's so hard to face the future. It's about being a warrior... this woman is acting as a warrior. That's the message and that's the lesson. Sometimes the hardest perspectives to see are plainly visible, if our eyes are open to it.

INSIGHT: A WARRIOR'S WAY

Dealing with your cancer diagnosis and thinking about having cancer are the scariest things most of us will ever face. Just when you think you have it tough, you learn of someone else in an even worse situation. Real survivors always keep things in perspective, recognizing that one's own predicament may seem incredibly easy or hopelessly difficult compared to somebody else's. Accept what you have — it's all you have. But always keep a larger perspective than just your own experience. It will help you to stay grounded, and to be wiser. Keep the courage to see that perspective.

CHAPTER TWENTY-SEVEN:
MY MOST IMPORTANT JOB
IS FIGHTING CANCER

Cancer patients and survivors not only have to battle the most horrible of diseases, but they usually must do so in the workplace, with everybody watching. I recall when virtually all of my hair fell out over one weekend — it bothered some people more than it bothered me... but then, I didn't have to look at my bright, bald, head. When cancer patients mix battling cancer with workplace demands a strange combination of joy and pain emerges.

We experience joy because we can still function, be with non-cancerous people, trying to act and be normal and focus on other challenges and concerns than the battle inside our bodies. The pain part is usually associated with our fatigue, our inability to think and remember effectively while striving to do well in our work.

Careers define our meaningfulness beyond selling our labor in the market. For some of us, it defines our purpose, the "footprint" of how we want to make our contribution. Sadly, for others, it's simply a place to exchange labor for money, without much personal satisfaction.

Fortunately for me, my work and my professional contributions are an extension of my spirit, an expression of who I am and what I value. My work brings me satisfaction and a sense of fulfillment, but it doesn't replace my identity, it only helps shape it. Living on purpose molds my identity daily.

Sadly but true, our careers — and our lives, depending on your viewpoint — are defined by the external world we live in. In this world, we still are defined as what we do, our job title or which company we work for.

As a cancer survivor, I have gradually learned to redefine my worth from external values, such as what the marketplace pays me, or whom I report to or what my professional credentials are. I now define my worth as knowing that my efforts make a difference... that I, John Cope, make a difference. I want my contributions to make a difference in the success of the enterprise and to have a positive impact on my colleagues. Of course, I still keep a scorecard of how I am recognized and rewarded for my efforts. I still want to make more money (who doesn't?), but internal satisfaction is more important than climbing the corporate ladder for the sake of external success.

The bottom line is that doing good work is much more important to me than recognition, promotions or other typical means of workplace validation.

As a cancer patient, my career took a back seat to my number one priority, fighting cancer. As a cancer survivor, my work, while still important, is relegated to a different priority than it previously was. Today, staying healthy and cancer-free is my primary job.

The world of work has its share of highs and lows, but nothing has taken me up and down the roller coaster of life faster than one day in cancer treatment. It's a wake-up call I will not forget.

Whether you are battling cancer or are a survivor, you know what is the worst thing that could happen to you. What's the worst thing that can happen to an employed person... losing a job? What a catastrophe — having to get another job! Try getting another life — now, that's a tough challenge!

Cancer survivors will understand this. When you face cancer and beat cancer and are a successful living survivor, the threat of losing a job is like losing your pocket change in a parking meter. It's simply no big deal. Admittedly, losing your job often means losing your medical benefits, which can be a big deal in the financial toll it can take on a family. However, you can always get another job. Lose the battle with cancer and it's pretty tough to get a new life.

Before I left the corporate world, my company was undergoing a major restructuring. Many people would be changing jobs, some losing their long-time positions, and yet other opportunities would be opening up. Workplace changes always bring both opportunity and threats. Each of us must decide how we interpret the changes, as threats or opportunities.

In my company's restructuring, the most senior officer I had reported to was retiring. The company had appointed a new president, an individual I had worked with in the past and respected a great deal. As the reconfiguration unfolded, it became clear that my own position was being put on the line. Either I would have a new job, possibly as a vice-president, or I'd be out the door with the tag line, "pursuing other opportunities." Only time would tell.

My staff was concerned about politics, that the VP role might not go to me for my contributions and potential, but to someone else for political reasons. My spouse and I discussed the risks, the potential outcomes, the professional goals I had set and decided, whatever the outcome, I and ultimately we, as a couple, would be fine. Though I would love the opportunity and challenge of being vice-president, if it didn't happen, it didn't happen.

What's the worst that could happen to a three-time cancer survivor...lose my job?

When it was announced that another individual was named vice-president, but that I was asked to be part of the organization in a different leadership role, a colleague approached me with concern. "I heard the news," he said. "This must be the most horrible day of your life. I am so sorry."

I looked him in the eye and replied, "No, this is not the worst day in my life, it's not even close! Being told you have cancer again, now that's a bad day." He smiled as if he understood, but he really didn't. That was okay, because I understand the difference and it's all that matters.

INSIGHT: A WARRIOR'S WAY

When you experience the perspective of being a cancer survivor, few events in your life matter as much as living life to the fullest. Lose a job? Sell the house? Relocate your family to a new city? Each of these events can bring significant changes, but they can't hold a candle to battling and beating cancer. Keep your perspective and priorities clear. They will guide you through the whitewater of changes you will face, in your career and in your life.

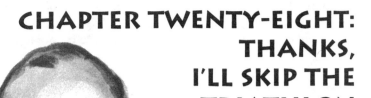

CHAPTER TWENTY-EIGHT: THANKS, I'LL SKIP THE TRIATHLON THIS YEAR

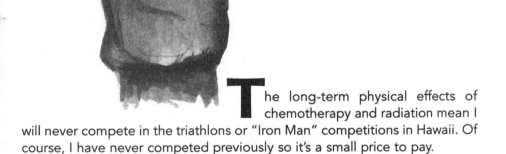

The long-term physical effects of chemotherapy and radiation mean I will never compete in the triathlons or "Iron Man" competitions in Hawaii. Of course, I have never competed previously so it's a small price to pay.

One of my greatest fears was that I would lose the athletic prowess that has given me endless hours of fun and healthy competition. I have also been proud of my coordination and natural athleticism. For many years, it was a significant part of my identity. Of course, the natural aging process slows us down and robs us of our youthful abilities; so at some point all of us must learn how to gently let go of our youthful strengths and abilities.

Chemotherapy and radiation change you in a right now, in your face, don't even try to argue with the changes that are happening kind of way. You're lucky to be alive, let alone hitting homeruns or beating your opponent forty-love. But it's not fair, your brain keeps reminding you. Other people can grow old gracefully and yet the ravages of the cure, to be able to live, take it away from you!

Accepting the unacceptable is what makes a warrior win. It's not what I would have chosen, but it's my reality. It's not the end of the world that I can't run like I used to... no. It's not the end of the world that I don't have the stamina that I expected... no. It's not the end of the world that I simply can't do the physical things I used to... no. Would I change it if I could? You bet. In a heartbeat! But I can't...

The harsh reality is that cancer changes you in unexpected and unwanted ways. Perhaps I have lost some physical abilities, but I have gained in the spiritual and emotional arenas in ways I could not have anticipated. In fact, I think having and fighting cancer have changed me in many ways, virtually all for the better, despite the pain and agony of the journey.

Attitude is key here. We change, we evolve, we all become different. The real question is, Do you see the glass as half empty or half full? Cancer survivors always see, or at least try to see, the glass as half full. We realize that although we give up some things in life, like our natural athleticism, we also open ourselves up to the importance of growing our spirit.

The attitude of successful warriors and cancer survivors is that we make our own choices and ultimately determine our destinies. I am choosing to not lose the battle with cancer... and they say the triathlon and Iron Man marathons are tough. Try beating cancer, baby!

INSIGHT: A WARRIOR'S WAY

The determination to battle and beat cancer is the warrior's way. Iron Man marathons and triathlons are for wimps, by comparison. Strive, every day, to have a warrior's attitude and you'll be a warrior and ultimately, control your own destiny. Oh, and one more thing — keep your attitude, it looks good on you!

CHAPTER TWENTY-NINE: REFLECTIONS WITH MY GREATEST CHAMPION, MY KELLY JO

Dealing with cancer has taught me many things, but one of the greatest surprises is to feel the joy in the flow of my own tears. These moments usually happen with the playing of the National Anthem or the sight of a small child, bald from chemotherapy and struggling to be happy, but once in awhile that joy comes from reflecting on my own experiences. I view these moments as a window into my soul. They allow me to test my behavior and thinking with what I am feeling and what is coming from the spirit within me. Am I truly behaving consistently with my values and purpose?

One June evening in 1999, in Jasper National Park, Kelly and I had finished dinner after a day of playing tourist. We were discussing future paths my professional career might take when, like many times before, a simple question brought my deepest thoughts surging to the surface. Here are those reflections.

"My fists are clenched as hard as I can make them. I feel passion, anger, intensity of emotion and a dogged determination to tell my story and help others adopt an attitude of being a survivor. Why? I am not ready to die. I want to experience more days like today, I want more of life, I want more of everything I haven't experienced yet.

"I have much to do yet in my life. I don't want others to live in fear. I am not afraid of cancer or of dying. But I am afraid that beyond all my efforts, all my determination, all my absolute resolve to live and living on purpose, cancer will come along again and bang! I'll be gone and it will be way too soon.

"I am a realist. I'll face cancer again. I am prepared for it. It's a battle I live everyday. The cancer "bugs" are running around in me... they never leave and I know that. That's just the way it is. Reality gives me the strength, the ability to accept what's in front of me. I know I can't do anything about having cancer, I can't make it go away and I can't deny I have fought and beaten cancer three times. I am living my life on purpose, as much as I can. In the big picture of things, I simply have to accept the reality of my situation and make the most of my life and shape my life with an attitude of "I AM A SURVIVOR!

"When I am in one of these reflective moods, my feelings of vulnerability, the feelings I have every day, rise to the surface and my tears just bubble up and out. Hell, I have hot flashes, lower intestinal problems and other painful symptoms of being a cancer survivor every day, but in my consciousness, I never forget I could be gone... Good Bye! I don't want that. I refuse to! I refuse to die!

"I am who I am. My attitude is who I am. It's who I have always been. I am strong and I know that. It's how I have survived. I have had an experience, battling cancer three times, that very few people have had. I didn't ask for this, God knows. But I have the courage to face the reality of my little world.

"I am not striving for perfection in my world — perfection isn't really possible. I haven't perfected living on purpose and I am certainly not a saint, far from it. Having had and surviving cancer never, never, leaves your consciousness. There's always a little voice that says, "John Cope, you will face cancer number four... that's the way it is."

My wife and I have a word, a term we have invented on this trip, to describe our feelings about log homes, those wonderful, huge, chalets or cabins that have walls with the thickness of huge timbers. We love them and someday, if I live long enough (there's that damn reality kicking in again), we will live in one of our own design. They symbolize much to us... heart, strength, stability, safety, all of the positive characteristics a house can be. We refer to this phenomenon as "Green Roof Envy," since the log homes we find ourselves 'oohing and aaahhing' and sighing over have a forest green roof and shiny brown log exterior.

"Green Roof Envy, yes, I want to have that experience and I am afraid I'll die before I can, which makes me all the more determined to live my life on purpose and achieve that vision. I want to be here, I want to be a survivor, I want to walk along the river, get smoke from the fire in my eyes, I want to be 75 years old with you and share that Green Roof Envy Log House with you.

"The first time I had cancer, I considered it a fluke, a freak accident. The second time, it almost took me away — the tumors wouldn't die. The third time I simply refused to allow cancer to take me away. I was going to win. I hope I will never have cancer again but I live my life on purpose, to make decisions that affect my life because I can... at least I can do that. But I have already faced cancer again, even after living my life on purpose, so is it really a great philosophy?"

"So, I had this little cough that wouldn't go away, a little lung problem, so I couldn't breathe, so what's the big deal. Same type of cancer but different this time. Every time I have had cancer, the cancer changed, but my attitude didn't change. I am going to beat this SOB!

"I think about doing something different, something to help people. I don't want them, other cancer survivors, to live in fear. Living in fear is NOT the way to live out the rest of your life. Cancer survivors, however, always live in the unknown, which often is labeled as fear. People should not live in fear of their career situations any more than they live with fear of dying. We need to make choices about who we are, what we do, how we want to live out our lives, and I want to share the "Kick Ass Spirit" in me. I want to share that... how do I do that? I want the 'Spirit' to live, I want that from deep in my gut!

"I have this image in my mind, a 'picture' frozen in time. It was in August, 1992, and I remember it was about not getting sunburned. Because of the chemotherapy drugs, I was vulnerable. It was a hot sun, and the drapes were drawn to block out the late afternoon heat. I remember so vividly my reality: one tumor gone, 'chemo'd' away, but the one remaining wouldn't go, it was stubborn, it wouldn't leave, it wouldn't die. Will I live, or will this be it? Enough questions to fill two or three Jeopardy television programs.

"I remember us touching, loving, hugging (as we are at this moment), wondering if I was going to live. That was a very telling moment in my life. In many ways it was a turning point in how I was going to face the realities of my cancerous body. There was and is a spirit between you and me.

I remember thinking that you and I might not have any say in what happens to me...to us.

"Chemotherapy is the battle I may not win, but I am a hard-nosed SOB and I can deal with the tough crap. I can deal with it again and I expect I will, but I may not prevail. But it won't be for lack of trying to control my destiny.

"I can do everything I can to be a successful survivor. A successful thriver! But I always know the fourth time may take me out permanently. No matter how much I fight and how much I want to do something different, it may not happen. That is the way of life, which is the way of reality.

"In some ways, it's like my little voice says, John, you're going to die. Blow the investments? Whatever. Save for retirement? You'll never get there. Return on your IRAs and 401K? It doesn't matter. But yet, I still have to believe I have a future. If a doctor were to tell me, Mr. Cope, you have "X" amount of time to live, I would say 'Screw You!' I won't accept that, you can never accept that diagnosis. That's what the spirit or fight is all about, it's not about denial, it's about facing the reality of each situation and having the courage to fight to control our destiny, in spite of the odds.

"The fight is all about being resilient against the fears and tugs of what might be. I would like to help people fight their own demons. When I soul search, in a very humble way, I don't believe I can help anybody, any cancer survivor at all. All I can hope for is to inspire them to find their own courage, deal with their own evils and commit to being a thriving survivor. It's the only way to live."

INSIGHT: A WARRIOR'S WAY

Moments of honest reflection, though sometimes emotionally draining, sometimes emotionally exhilarating, are always insightful and always lead to strength and courage. Find ways to talk about your innermost thoughts, your innermost demons and your innermost passions with someone you love. You'll both be richer for it. I know I have been enriched by my efforts to live according to my values and my beliefs, but probably most importantly, to share my life with my greatest champion. Thank you, Kelly Jo. I love you.

ABOUT THE AUTHOR

JOHN R. COPE

John R. Cope is a professional speaker, author, and a three-time breast cancer survivor who lives in Lake Oswego, Oregon.

Just before his 40th birthday John was diagnosed with breast cancer. After his mastectomy and six months of chemotherapy, his life returned to normal. He believed his battle with breast cancer was won.

Less than five years later, his breast cancer returned. During six months of intensive chemotherapy, his prognosis remained questionable. In spite of overwhelming odds, he beat cancer a second time.

About four years later, John was once again diagnosed with breast cancer. After three months of radiation his cancer is back in remission.

The odds of a male having breast cancer even once are astronomical. There are better odds of winning the lottery and being hit by lighting on the same day.

After a career in corporate America, John is president of his own management consulting firm, John Cope and Associates. Prior to founding his own firm, he held executive management positions in high-technology firms and the public sector. He began his professional career as a jail psychologist. He is a board member of a privately held company and is a charter member of the California Career Development Futures Forum.

A dynamic public speaker, he combines humor with the honesty only a three-time cancer survivor can have. His newest book, A Warrior's Way: Insights for Cancer Patients, Cancer Survivors and Those Who Love Them, is a collection of vignettes gleaned from his three battles with cancer. Told with a sometimes serious approach but sprinkled with a strong dose of humor, his story is a triumph of hope and courage.

Contact him at (503) 638-1611 or toll free at 1 (877) 638-1686 or fax (503) 638-6962 or by email at john@johncope.com

HEARTS THAT CARE PUBLISHING™ ORDER FORM

	Quantity	Price at $12.95ea. (U.S.)
A Warrior's Way: Insights for Cancer Patients, Cancer Survivors and Those Who Love Them©		
Shipping and Handling (see chart below)		
Subtotal		
($12.95 U.S. / $18.95 Canada) **Total Amount**		

Shipping Information
Shipping and Handling

Quantity ordered:	Please Add:
1-2	$3.50
3-4	$5.50
5-6	$7.50

Call for quotes on quantity orders

Please make checks payable to
Hearts That Care Publishing
51 Hillshire Drive,
Lake Oswego, Oregon 97034-7375

Call Toll Free to Order: 1-877-638-1686
EMAIL orders to: Bookorder@johncope.com
(www:johncope.com)
FAX orders to: 503.638.6962

Method of Payment
☐ Enclosed is my check or money order

Please charge to:
☐ MasterCard ☐ VISA ☐ American Express ☐ Discover

Credit Card account number _____

Expiration Date: _____/_____ Signature:_____

Name as it appears on credit card:_____

Ship-To Address

_____
Name

_____
Company

_____
Address

_____
City   State   Zip

_____
E-mail address

_____
Day Phone Number (should we need to contact you)